THIRD SPACE
BOLTON

A STORY ABOUT SUPPORTING YOUNG PEOPLE TODAY

MARK COWLING

ISBN: **1729784127**
ISBN-13: **978-1729784129**

DEDICATION

Thanks to Julian, Steve, Moira, Penny and Matt.

And to the team:
Julie, Guy, Chris, Lily Jo
and some incredible volunteers.

CONTENTS

Things are different today

Teenagers spend an average of nine hours a day online locked on to mobile phones. Social media is shaping young people far more dramatically than television has ever done. And because it starts well before the teenage years, some argue that youth work with teenagers is too late to make a difference to the formation of young people.

Since time immemorial things have been changing. People explore, discover, develop and make. As a result, the way we do things changes. But being creatures of habit, most human beings struggle with change more and more, the longer and longer they get used to one way of doing things. Each generation has been challenged by an ever-accelerating pace of change in our world. In recent years we seen some really big shifts that have been described as changes from modernity to postmodernity, from the industrial age to the information age, from Christendom to post-Christendom, from production to consumerism, and from religious identity to spiritual exploration. Young people are full citizens of the present.

The World Health Organisation (WHO) definition of Health is a "state of complete physical, mental and social well-being and not merely the absence of disease or infirmity." This definition of health is key to quality of life and transcends standard of living, another WHO measurement of wellbeing. But, such dramatic and fast paced change has created new challenges for our wellbeing today. The story of Third Space Bolton is our experience of these challenges and our learning about how to support, inspire and unite young people to improve their wellbeing in our changing world.

Third space is a sociological term used to describe leisure time. It's a space that is actually really important for people as it provides a time to rest and reflect on all of life, including your first space which is your family time and your second space, which is your work time. Third Space Bolton aims to be a resource for young people in their third space. We particularly want to support learning and the putting into practice of skills for wellbeing for the whole of life.

Obstacles to wellbeing

Wellbeing in teenagers is affected by a number of things: Firstly, there are your genes, passed down from your parents, which will affect the probability of suffering from depression for example. Secondly, hormones. These are literally raging in the body of a teenager, released for physiological development but affecting the emotions. Thirdly, circumstances affect our wellbeing, especially when you have no experiential history to help you. When all three factors come together, you're chance of suffering ill health affecting emotional wellbeing are greatly increased.

Another major factor in teenagers is their brains. Rob Parsons (Care for the Family) puts it like this:

"We used to think the brain was fully developed by late childhood. We always knew there was a burst of brain activity around toddlerhood, but what they discovered is there a similar burst of brain growth around puberty. But, whereas around toddlerhood it's around balance and movement, around puberty, it's about emotion and memory. If being around your teenage daughter is like sitting at the feet of an emotional volcano, you're not far from the mark. If you've ever said to your teenager "you're behaving like a two year old", again you're not that

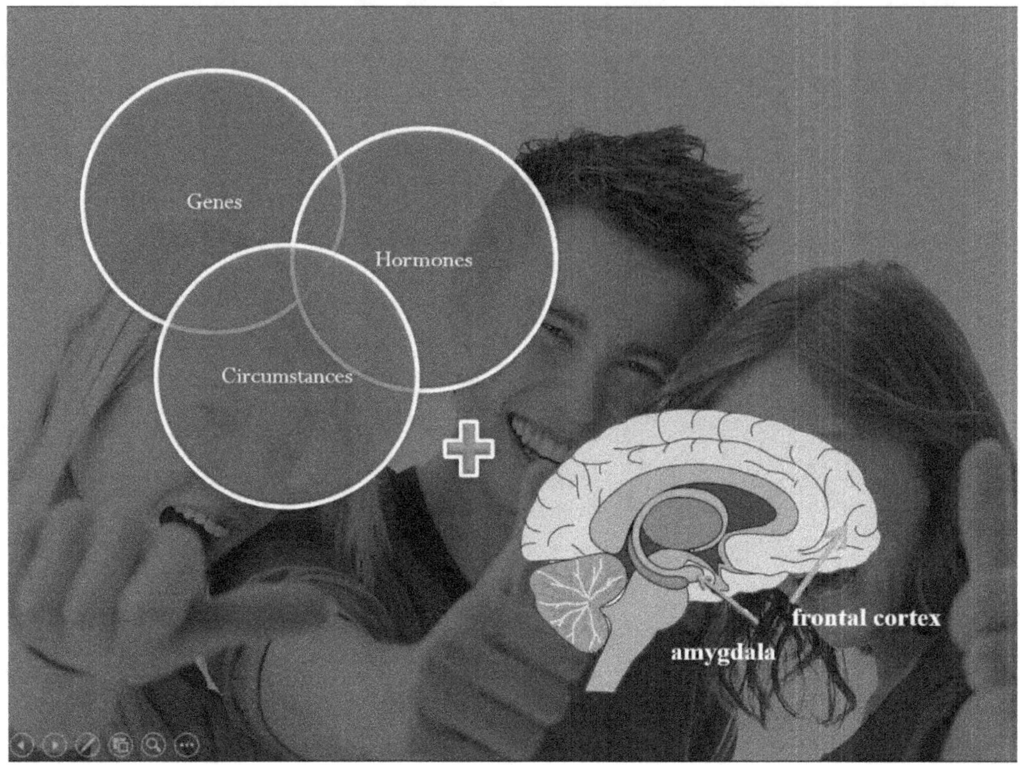

far off the mark. But the last bit to develop is at the pre-frontal cortex and it's the bit of the brain psychologists call the brain's policeman. Some call it the brakes. It's the bit of the brain that gives you sound judgement. That bit of the brain is still developing, so we say "how can you think of skateboarding of a twenty foot high wall. Why didn't you put your seat belt on. That bit of the brain is still growing. It's the bit of the brain for example that allows you to defer immediate gratification for the sake of longer term good. We say "How can you think of going clubbing the night before your GCSE maths exam for goodness sake?" "Dad, the exam isn't until tomorrow afternoon for goodness sake!" That bit of the brain is still developing. And that's why it's important to just get our teenagers through. Just hang in there with them. They are literally a work in progress. The scary thing is one psychologist said some teenagers don't get their brakes until they're twenty-five years old. And certainly that's true."

Teenager's brains are dealing with new experiences of emotions and to that extent they do it from a place of experiential blindness. By way of illustration of experiential blindness, take a look at the image of black and white blobs to see if you can see any pattern or picture. Then go to the back of this book and look at the higher definition version of this picture. It will "heal" your experiential blindness so that now when you look at the black and white blobs picture you will see a pattern or image. The brain sifts through past experiences and when there's new knowledge there it changes the way you experience these blobs. It's the same principle with emotions. Neuroscientists call these "predictions" making sense of the world and it means that feelings are a physiology that need to be translated into emotions. That translation is a process that enables emotions to be analysed, controlled and influenced.

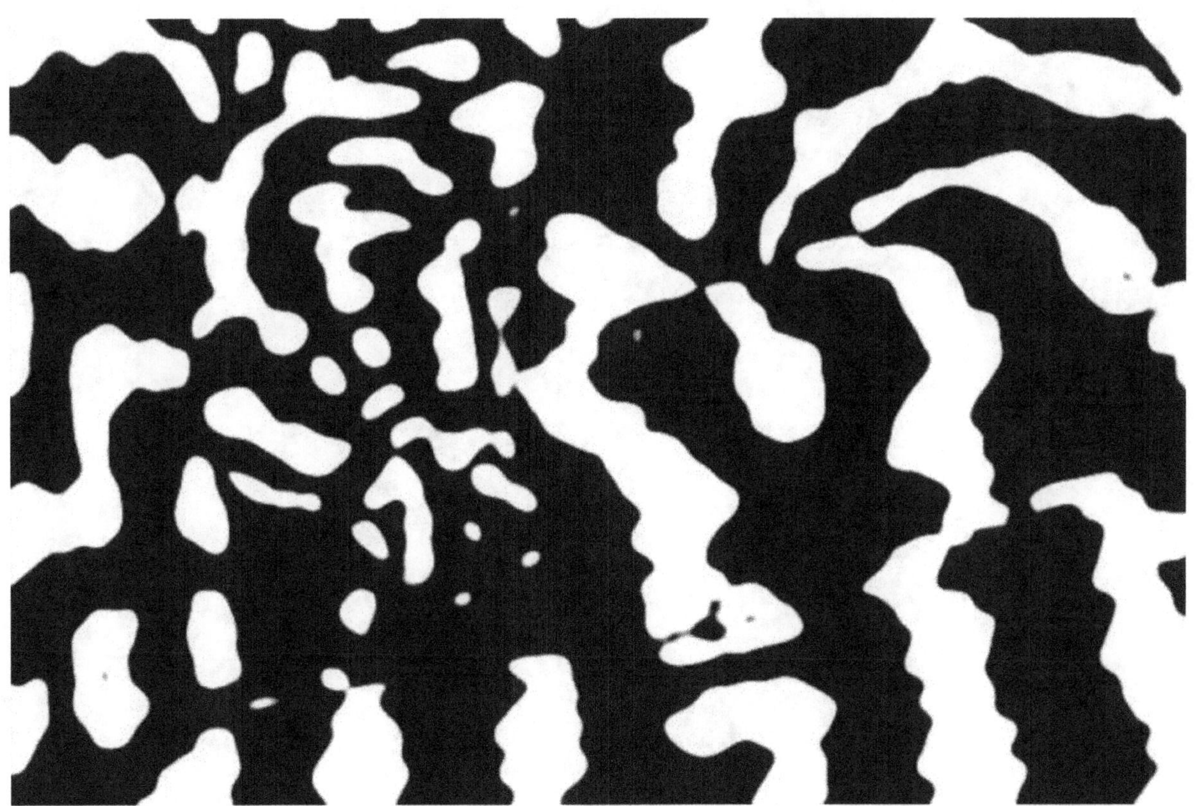

Adolescents need third space

And this takes us to the final factor that affects wellbeing of teenagers: **Coaching** is the extra factor. Coaching is defined as "a form of development supporting a learner in achieving a specific personal or professional goal by providing training and guidance."

Rob Parsons (Care for the Family) puts it like this:

"You know sometimes we are so busy looking for academic or sporting success we forget to commend character. I remember when my son Lloyd was seventeen and had passed his driving test. He bought an old jalopy motor car. He came home one night and he said "Dad, I was down the road and I saw this old lady and she looked lost. And I said "Are you alright my dear?" "No," she said, "son, I'm lost," "Well, I've got a car, I'll take you home." And he said "Dad I took her right to her front door and she said "This is not my house." And I said "Well where is your house?" And she gave me another address and I took her there and she said "This is not my house." And he said "Dad, I took her to six other houses. And finally, I took her to a police station." And he's seventeen, and he's driving me crazy and his bedroom's a mess and I have to drag him out of bed for school and I've just caught him smoking. But he said to an old lady "My dear, can I help you?" I have to commend that. This is character."

The best coaches in the world are parents because no-one knows their child like they do and no-one loves their child like they do. Experts have boiled down some of the foundations to good parenting.

1.) Family provides **support, a moral compass, a place to learn & relate. Play and fun** is essential for child development.

2.) Love is spelt **T-I-M-E** and we need to prioritise and plan our time with our children. Children thrive on **routine**

3.) Self confidence and wellbeing are received through **love languages** such as Affirming words; Affectionate touch; 1to1 Time; Thoughtful presents; Kind actions

4.) Setting **authoritative** boundaries that combine a **warm** but **firm** style is ideal. Choosing the right battles helps when we recognise "**HALT**" (Hungry, Angry, Lonely, Tired)

5.) Model relationships with active listening; paying full attention, showing interest, reflecting back, supporting sibling relationships; helping manage anger and resolve conflict

6.) Training for **healthy independence;** avoiding over-control, Helping children make good choices; inc. sex, internet, drugs & alcohol, Passing on beliefs and values through discussion with family and other role models.

Third Space is a sociological term used to describe leisure time. First space is family time and second space is your work time. Third space is really important for people as it provides a time to rest and reflect on all of life – a place to be coached.   Third Space Bolton wants to support young people by resourcing this space.

BABY

CHILD

ADOLESCENT

YOUNG ADULT

PARENT

GRANDPARENT

Adolescence is the third of six life stages and it needs support because it drastically affects the next life stages. 50% of mental health problems are established by age fourteen; 75% by the early twenties. It's also a strongly self-conscious stage, where talking about challenges and change is hard to do. For example, 70% of teens hide their online usage from their parents. The African proverb "it takes a village to raise child" recognises that we all need to do our bit bringing up young people. It also understands that often parents are perceived by their children as being too close to open up to. With family fragmentation also a common reality today, schools have recognised that support from outside the family is vital. But schools also acknowledge their limitations; measures are weighted to academic results which relegates resources given to developing wellbeing and many teachers are not keen to accept an additional social care responsibility. Cuts to health and social services mean professionals in the community are only scratching the surface of need. When faced with the need today, there is a crisis in support for young people's wellbeing.

Coaching is a form of early intervention which passes on skills to help the individual but also to equip people to pastorally care for others in a team or family setting. The suicide statistics on page 15 show that men don't talk. But coaching in our experience, transforms this situation, creating men who are champions for getting other men to talk. Empathy is a key skill in coaching. The same can be true for young people.

Brene Brown (Researcher and Author) explains the importance of empathy over sympathy:

"So what is empathy, and why is it very different than sympathy? Empathy fuels connection. Sympathy drives

disconnection. Empathy, it's very interesting. Teresa Wiseman is a nursing scholar who studied professions – very diverse professions – where empathy is relevant and came up with four qualities of empathy – perspective taking, the ability to take the perspective of another person or recognise their perspective as their truth, staying out of judgement – not easy when you enjoy it as much as most of us do – recognising emotion in other people, and then communicating that. Empathy is feeling with people. And to me, I always think of empathy as this kind of sacred space when someone is kind of in a deep hole, and they shout out from the bottom and they say, I'm stuck. It's dark. I'm overwhelmed. And then we look and we say, hey, I'm down. I know what it's like down here, and you're not alone. Sympathy is, oh, it's bad, uh-huh. No. Do you want a sandwich? Empathy is a choice, and it's a vulnerable choice. Because in order to connect with you, I have to connect with something in myself that knows that feeling. Rarely, if ever, does an empathic response begin with 'at least'. I had a – yeah. And we do it all the time. Because you know what? Someone just shared something with us that's incredibly painful, and we're trying to silver lining it. I don't think that's a verb, but I'm using it as one. We're trying to put the silver lining around it. So I had a miscarriage. Oh, at least you know you can get pregnant. I think my marriage is falling apart. At least you have a marriage, John's getting kicked out of school. At least Sarah is an A student. But one of the things we do sometimes in the face of very difficult conversations is we try to make things better. If I share something you that's very difficult, I'd rather you say I don't even know what to say right now. I'm just so glad you told me. Because the truth is rarely can a response make something better. What makes something better is connection."

Third Space Bolton, founded by local Christian leaders, could see a skilled resource already in the community that could be used to make a bigger impact in coaching. Church youth workers, who lead and resource their own third space activities in churches, are often experienced young adults with the right skills to reach adolescents. Many of them also have their finger on the pulse of social, cultural and spiritual changes in our communities. For example, they are aware of four highly prevalent "post-Christian" beliefs of teenagers today;

    1.) **Identity: being true to yourself and doing what's right for you.**

Whilst this can empower the minority in a positive way, it also elevates ourselves above what's good for others. It supposes our judgements are the best, elevating us to God.

2.) **Freedom: being free to do what you want so long as it's not harming someone else.**

Whilst this respects the rights of individuals it can negate the responsibilities of individuals and of wellbeing.

3.) **Happiness: believing you've got to do what makes you happy in the end.**

The Christian tradition has shown that when we aim for righteousness (wellbeing *or shalom*) we get blessedness (happiness), but when we aim for blessedness we get neither blessedness nor righteousness.   Brene   Brown,   discussing   her   research,   puts   it   like   this; *"Let me tell you what we think about children. They're hardwired for struggle when they get here. And when you hold those perfect little babies in your hand, our job is not to say, "Look at her, she's perfect. My job is just to keep her perfect — make sure she makes the tennis team by fifth grade and Yale by seventh grade." That's not our job. Our job is to look and say, "You know what? You're imperfect, and you're wired for struggle, but you are worthy of love and belonging." That's our job. Show me a generation of kids raised like that, and we'll end the problems I think that we see today."*

4.) **Morality: believing no-one has the right to tell anyone else what's wrong or right for someone else.**

Whilst this respects human rights and dignity, it again, can lead to outcomes for individuals and communities that do not benefit wellbeing. For example, there's a huge amount of content accessed by young people on Youtube that is sensational, not real nor good advice. Historically, religious debate involved deciding my religion is true and yours is untrue. Today, the claim that salvation has been revealed in one religion (a better way) is considered evil by a growing number in our society.

Social wellbeing

Teenagers encounter obstacles to their **social wellbeing**. Everybody experiences important relationships deteriorating around them:

- 50% families experience a parental split

- 50% people who leave a job do so because of a poor relationship with their boss

- One in three university students experiences sexual abuse

Whilst an ideology of wall dismantling was prominent in the 1980s (Berlin wall), today there is more wall building (Trump's Mexico border and Brexit). As tensions grow, there is a growing need for peace-making skills at every level of society, starting with ourselves.

The online world is creating problems for people. The prevalence of online gambling advertising has led to the number of problem gamblers growing by a third in three years to nearly half a million people. Men age 12-17 are the biggest users of online porn which experts say has caused an "adjusting of what is normal". 83% of men have watched porn by age 18 with 66% secretive about it with parents. A new online culture of "Laddism" has emerged. For example the online site UniLad, which attracts male university students, is criticised for condoning the harming of women. Surveys reports that one third of university students are sexually assaulted highlighting a disregard of the law on the matter of consent. Statistics show sex assault overall has gone up 21% and rape by 29%, whereas other violent crime in total is down (despite a concerning spike in knife-crime amongst often, disadvantaged young people).

Emotional wellbeing

25% of young people suffer from clinically diagnosable **mental health**

problems:

- 8% teens suffer depression and anxiety

- 10% teens are self-harming -most starting at age twelve. A

    common cause is traumatic stress*.

- 7% of people will attempt suicide at some point in their life. It's

    the biggest killer of men under 40 in the UK and rates are going

    up.

- 78% of eleven – sixteen year olds in one survey said that they had been bereaved of a close relative or

    friend. At the time of writing, 23,600 parents died in the UK last year, leaving dependent children.

    Other causes of loss experienced; job loss in the family, loss of a girlfriend/boyfriend

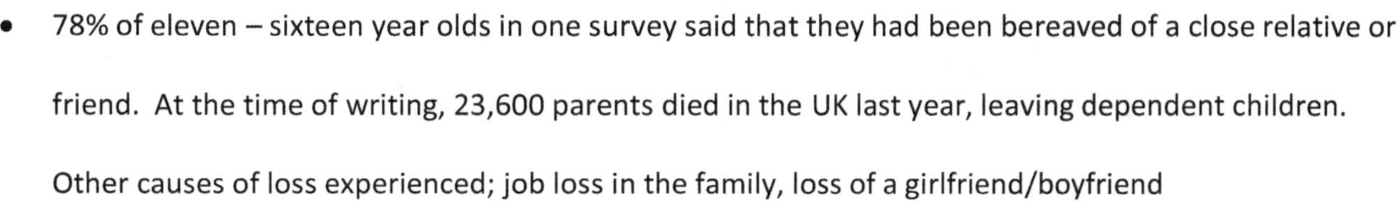

CAUSES OF TRAUMATIC STRESS ❖

1.) DIFFICULTIES AT HOME
2.) ARGUMENTS OR PROBLEMS
   WITH FRIENDS
3.) SCHOOL PRESSURES
4.) BULLYING
5.) DEPRESSION
6.) ANXIETY
7.) LOW SELF-ESTEEM
8.) TRANSITIONS AND CHANGES
   SUCH AS CHANGING SCHOOLS
9.) ALCOHOL AND DRUG USAGE.

Emotional health is not just about dealing with the crisis. It's also about building emotional intelligence (EI) -the capacity to manage your emotions. Research shows that EI has a cash value. EI improves mental health, job performance, leadership, social bonds and life balance. EI relates better to diversity, which builds cohesion.

Although EI is caught from role models rather than taught, the acronym RULER provides five steps to coach EI: **R**ecognizing emotion, **U**nderstanding emotion, **L**abelling emotion, **E**xpressing emotion, and **R**egulating emotion.

Personality
Myers Briggs Type Indicator

Communication
5 love languages

Culture
The way we do things around here

Race
Segregation and Protest

Gender
Patriarchs, Feminism, Transgender

Sexuality
Heterosexual-LGBT-Friendships

Religion
God-Science-Secularism

Able Bodied
Physical and Emotional Health

Physical wellbeing

Teenagers also encounter obstacles to their **physical wellbeing**.

Behind everything we take into our bodies (alcohol, sugar, drugs), there is an individual narrative playing out, which is social, emotional and physical.

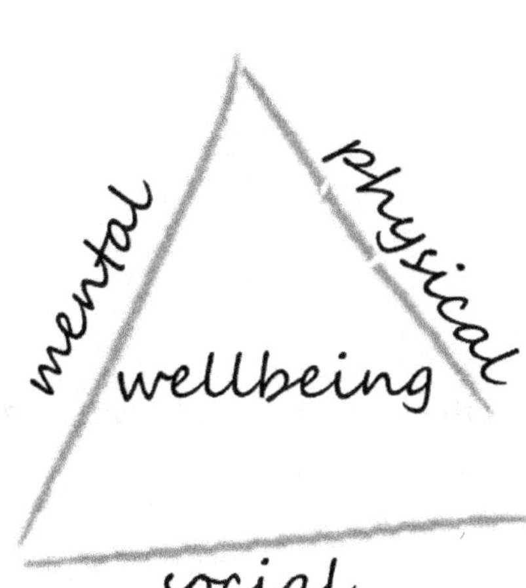

- 21% of teenagers are obese and 33% overweight or obese

- Harm from drug misuse means there is;

    o a 6-10% increase in deaths and hospitalisation per year.

    o 15% of pupils admit to having taken drugs

    o 6% of eleven year olds said they had tried drugs and 24% of 15 year olds.

Strong habits and addictions often trap us.

To catch a monkey, some African tribes put an orange inside a coconut and tie the coconut to a tree. There is a small hole in the coconut and when the monkey puts his hand inside to grab the orange, it cannot then pull its hand with the orange in it out. But because it doesn't want to let go of the orange, it is trapped.

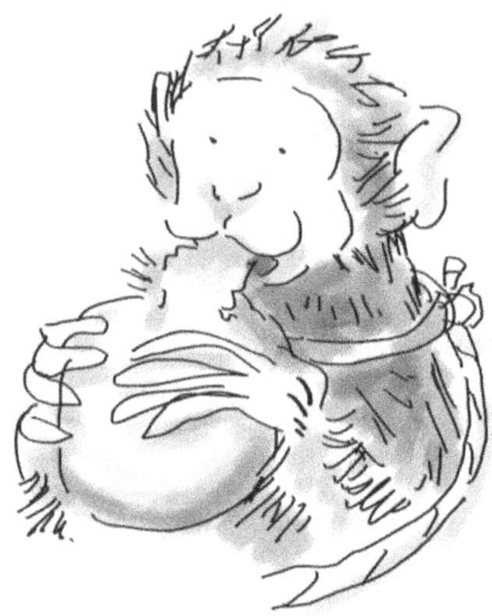

Like the monkey, we all have things in our lives that are like that orange and life involves learning to let go of these things. The four recommended steps to getting free from strong habits and addictions are:

1) Admitting – denial is the biggest obstacle to overcoming our unhelpful habits

2) Desiring to let go –agreeing that life without the "orange" in our life would be preferable

3) Planning boundaries –considering what boundaries need to be put in place to enable us to stay free

4) Setting gatekeepers –determining who we can be accountable to and supported by as we try to live with the boundaries

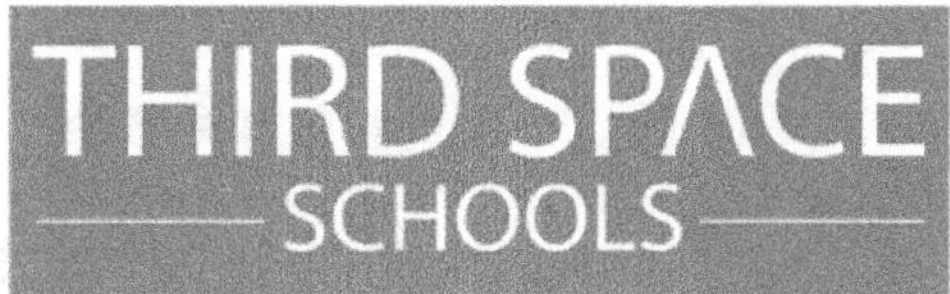

The Third Space Bolton curriculum offered for young people today supports and inspires social, emotional, physical and spiritual wellbeing.

Schools: Social wellbeing

Young people have a huge appetite for third space. Lunch clubs and after school sessions offering third space can be really popular. In a world where teenagers spend an average of nine hours a day online locked on to mobile phones, offering a real, not virtual, relational third space is a precious oasis for many.

In some cultures, third space is conducted around the fire pit or the water well. It's here in this transcendent setting the magic of third space is woven. Secrets of life are passed on from one generation to the next. It forms part of a rite of passage into adulthood, where young adults also learn about the challenges and responsibilities to their families and communities.

In a forty-five minute lunch club, we bring the rules of council from the fire pit into the classroom to capture something of the magic of the transcendent moment. Every member is invited to read out loud with personality, these rules, as part of their initiation into the group. When anyone speaks, they hold the Talking Stick, a physical reminder of their moment to speak and be listened to.

The rules of council (over the page) help ensure that nothing is unfair for anyone and that no-one gets in the way of another enjoying the session. It's rare that the discipline of young people following the rules of council becomes a problem. But in some challenging environments, we use a yellow and red card system to re-enforce the rules. Two yellow cards for rule breaking results in a red card and being asked to leave the "pitch" (session) for today. Leaving the session early results in a red card which also carries a ban for the next session. These boundaries become quickly respected and do protect the group from sabotage.

With this activity comes the chance to learn people's name and remember their story. It is the beginning of relationship and the journey of community which is often what the working day (second space) can squash out. We also start by going around the group, asking people to score how they feel today out of ten. And then to give us one word that describes why they scored themselves with that number. We need to discover, over the weeks, that it's normal to have ups and downs in how we feel about life, and to grow in confidence and purpose in sharing about that.

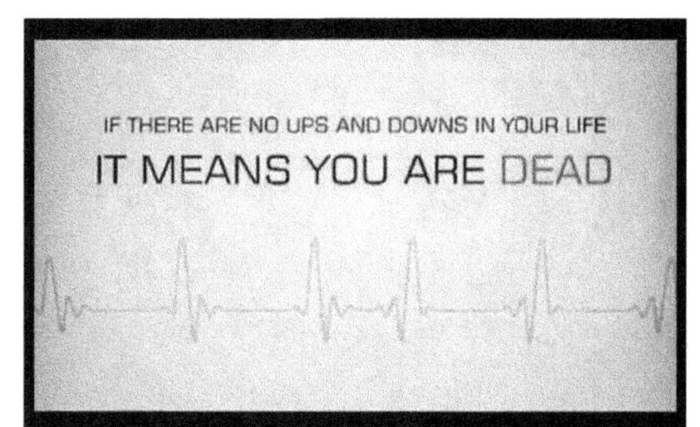

Mark Cowling (Third Space Bolton) puts it like this:

Amazingly, I ended up in the same industry as one of my high school friends -Mike. I worked for an international medical company and he worked for our biggest competitor. The business was famous for setting challenging sales targets and every month you saw where you stood on the company leader-board. Top achievement led to the glory of huge prizes and adoration at the national sales meetings. But we all knew poor results was a signal of poor performance and would leave us open to being pushed out of the company. We had a fantastic product that changed lives, but under this pressure, I found myself so focused on the sales numbers that I treated everybody like a transaction rather than a person. Would the stock room manager let me have the space I needed on her shelves? Would the surgeon choose to implant my product today? Once, when a patient had a cardiac arrest on the table, I was more concerned about getting the prosthesis implanted so I could charge the sale, than whether the patient lived or died! Everything I did and said had the goal of getting the right transaction from the person. Mike's career in his company took him to the very top, still in his thirties, where he reported directly to the President. He became a very wealthy man, sitting on the board of the company. I assumed that he played golf a lot with the President and must have become like a family member, running the big corporation. But, no. Mike recently told me he was just a number to the President, he had no depth of relationship with him and he felt he was very replaceable. The penny dropped. When we're under pressure we treat people like transactions. We do it at the supermarket to the checkout girl when we're in a rush and we do it when we feel the pressure of targets at work. It can even happen in the classroom at school -teachers can treat children like transactions, commodities to get results with. Resilience is needed in life to push back against these forces, to become more human and to enjoy more wellbeing in our lives. Third space is the place where we build resilience so we can go again. This is the essence of transcendent moments in life. A fire pit is optional.

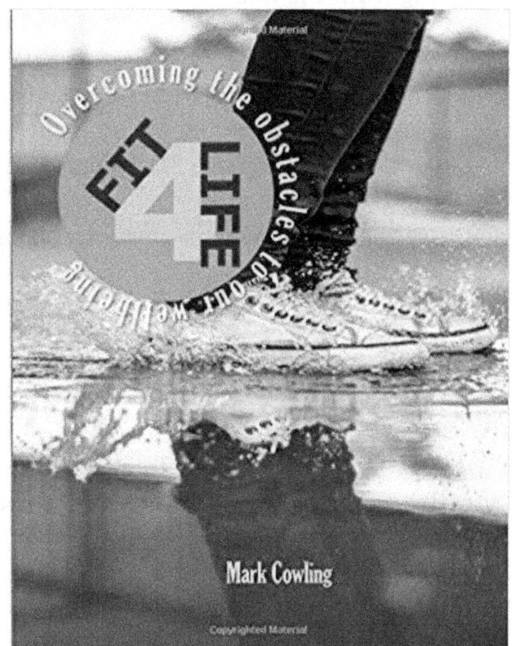

The Fit 4 Life Course covers 12 foundations which can help us overcome the opposing forces to our health and wellbeing. Learning about being fit and well can enable you to be "fit for life" but it can also help you to help others.

RULES OF COUNCIL

(S)HE WHO HOLDS THE TALKING STICK HOLDS

COUNCIL

"Speak what we feel, not what we ought to say"

–William Shakespeare, King Lear

Speaking from the heart

When speaking from the heart, we speak with simplicity and honesty. We aim to leave preconceived thoughts, ideas and concepts outside the circle letting the truth of the moment allow what needs to be said.

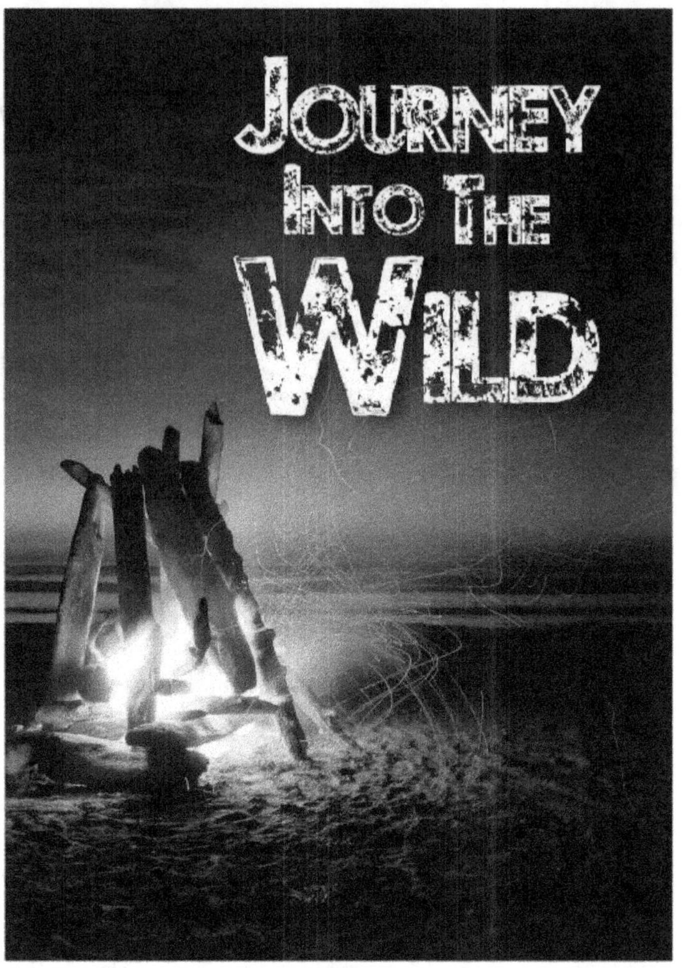

Listening from the heart

When practising listening from the heart we aim to leave judgements outside the circle. We listen with our whole body and being, like listening to the wind or the silence at dawn. When we listen this way we start to embrace the person who is speaking. When listening deeply we feel the connection of our truth with the truth of others.

Lean with words

We take collective responsibility for the time, knowing that if some people need more others will realise the need to take less.

Confidentiality

It is important to feel safe enough to share our heartfelt truths without the fear of gossip.

Consent

In a world where there are forces at work that de-humanise us, young people need to be informed about

consent.

The legal definition of consent is;

agreeing by

choice and having the

freedom and

capacity to make that

choice"

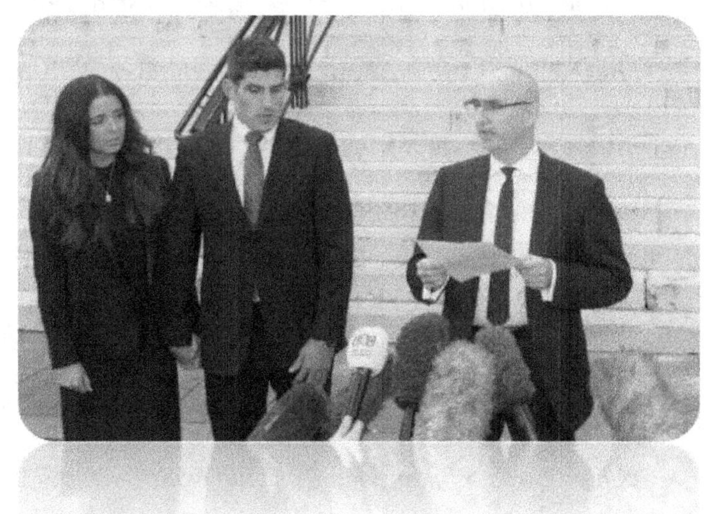

Ched Evans, a professional footballer had his career

derailed by a prosecution for rape. The case was

controversially quashed and a "not guilty" verdict was

given in the retrial when the sexual history of the woman

involved was admitted as evidence. Whatever the rights and wrongs in this case, it will further inhibit the coming forward of the 43% of victims who don't report sexual abuse.

Everybody needs to be aware today that CONSENT has no time limits. Operation Yew Tree, which investigated historic sexual abuse allegations, has shown that, what is done today can be prosecuted in fifty, sixty or seventy years time. The consequences to victims is long lasting. The damage to the reputation of perpetrators is costly. When the "brakes" aren't there in young people...there's a risk.

Third Space Bolton coaches teach young people about consent. We talk through graphic scenarios where we ask "how does this relate to the law, what does it say about the relationship and how did this happen?"

Consent: Not actually that complicated (by Blue Seat Studios).

If you're still struggling, just imagine instead of initiating sex, you're making them a cup of tea.

You say "hey, would you like a cup of tea?" and they go "omg yes, I would LOVE a cup of tea! Thank you!" then you know they want a cup of tea.*

If you say "hey, would you like a cup of tea?" and they um and ahh and say, "I'm not really sure..." then you can make them a cup of tea or not, but be aware that they might not drink it, and if they don't drink it then – this is the important bit – don't make them drink it. You can't blame them for you going to the effort of making the tea on the off-chance they wanted it; you just have to deal with them not drinking it. Just because you made it doesn't mean you are entitled to watch them drink it.

If they say "No thank you" then don't make them tea. At all. Don't make them tea, don't make them drink tea, don't get annoyed at them for not wanting tea. They just don't want tea, ok?

They might say "Yes please, that's kind of you" and then when the tea arrives they actually don't want the tea at all. Sure, that's kind of annoying as you've gone to the effort of making the tea, but they remain under no obligation to drink the tea. They did want tea, now they don't. Sometimes people change their mind in the time it takes to boil that kettle, brew the tea and add the milk. And it's ok for people to change their mind, and you are still not entitled to watch them drink it even though you went to the trouble of making it.

If they are unconscious, don't make them tea. Unconscious people don't want tea and can't answer the question "do you want tea" because they are unconscious.

Ok, maybe they were conscious when you asked them if they wanted tea, and they said yes, but in the time it took you to boil that kettle, brew the tea and add the milk they are now unconscious. You should just put the tea down, make sure the unconscious person is safe, and – this is the important bit – don't make them drink the tea. They said yes then, sure, but unconscious people don't want tea.

If someone said yes to tea, started drinking it, and then passed out before they'd finished it, don't keep on pouring it down their throat. Take the tea away and make sure they are safe. Because unconscious people don't want tea. Trust me on this.

If someone said "yes" to tea around your house last Saturday, that doesn't mean that they want you to make them tea all the time. They don't want you to come around unexpectedly to their place and make them tea and force them to drink it going "BUT YOU WANTED TEA LAST WEEK", or to wake up to find you pouring tea down their throat going "BUT YOU WANTED TEA LAST NIGHT".

Do you think this is a stupid analogy? Yes, you all know this already – of course you wouldn't force feed someone tea because they said yes to a cup last week. Of COURSE you wouldn't pour tea down the throat of an unconscious person because they said yes to tea five minutes ago when they were conscious. But if you can understand how completely ludicrous it is to force people to have tea when they don't want tea, and you are able to understand when people don't want tea, then how hard is it to understand when it comes to sex?

Whether it's tea or sex, Consent Is Everything. And on that note, I am going to make myself a cup of tea.

The subject of consent in relationships also requires an understanding about the power of emotions. Desire is one of the two most powerful emotions human beings experience -the other is anger. And our emotions can be manipulated by the images and behaviours projected on to us in the media and by our peers. This takes us onto the subject of emotional wellbeing.

Schools: Emotional wellbeing

In a world where 25% young people suffer from clinically diagnosable **mental health problems,** we need to offer support and encouragement to those facing crisis and to all who need to build life balance.

Stress is a good thing until it's a bad thing. Our genes, hormones and circumstances all contribute to stress affecting us negatively. We need to learn when stress is affecting a negatively and how to deal with it.

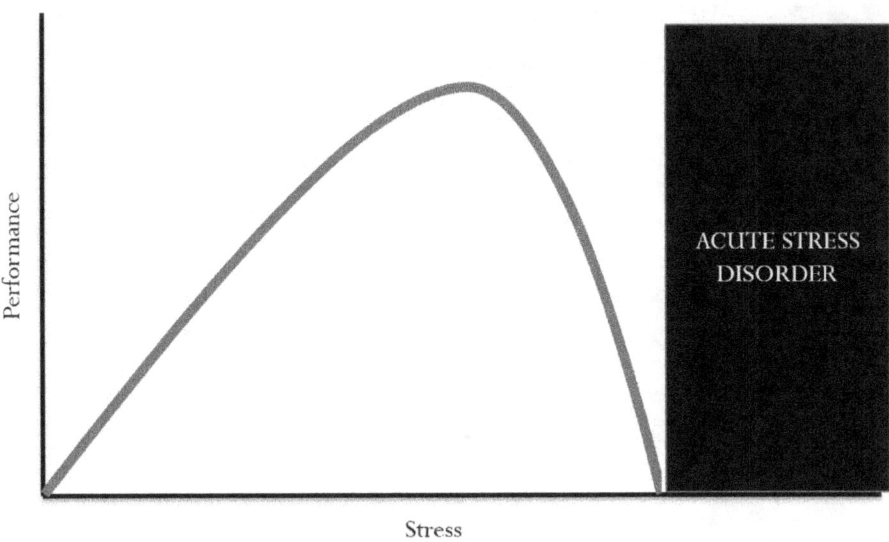

Research tells us the most common causes of stress which we need to learn to manage:

	Top Causes of Stress in the U.S.	Factors
1	Job Pressure	Co-Worker Tension, Bosses, Work Overload
2	Money	Loss of Job, Reduced Retirement, Medical Expenses
3	Health	Health Crisis, Terminal or Chronic Illness
4	Relationships	Divorce, Death of Spouse, Arguments with Friends, Loneliness
5	Poor Nutrition	Inadequate Nutrition, Caffeine, Processed Foods, Refined Sugars
6	Media Overload	Television, Radio, Internet, E-Mail, Social Networking
7	Sleep Deprivation	Inability to release adrenaline and other stress hormones

Third Space Bolton prioritises support for two common mental health issues and the associated tools for our emotional wellbeing toolbox.

- Anxiety

- Low Mood – Sadness, anxious or panicky, worry, tiredness, low self-esteem, frustration, anger

Third Space Bolton has partnered with thelilyjoproject.com to deliver teaching and coaching on these topics in high schools:

Tolu shares:

I suffered with clinical depression which I didn't realise I had at the time. My parents moved to the UK from Nigeria in the 80s and I was born in England. Everything was on a plate for me in life, until at university when I was twenty two I had a car crash. It was the first thing that had gone majorly wrong. That's quite late to have something that knocks you. I was kind of up on a pedestal and I didn't know how to deal with it. It knocked me out of uni for a few months which meant I had to resit my final year. A few other things began to happen at the same time that I tried to deal with on my own. Financial issues at home, a family member died, and a criminal accusation was made against me that was later proven false. I slowly curled up into a ball and left Manchester and tried to sort this out myself. The first step was realising something was wrong. I was so cut off, it was like being in a dark forest. I had no motivation and I just accepted that but then I saw a speck of light and realised staying in the dark wasn't where I was supposed to be. I started making connections with people on the outside. I had to stick my hand out to see if people would help me. And they did. I think now, it's important to realise we're all vulnerable and we need to do things to look after ourselves. Now I'm a full time musician which I never thought I would be, but I'm loving it.

Thinking negatively can spiral resulting in low mood. Negative thought styles to be aware of include;

Mind reading - Thinking you know what someone else is thinking – it's about you, and its negative. You end up reacting to what you *imagine* they are thinking.

Filtering - Seeing only the bad and ignoring the good eg Getting 90% in a mock test, and beating yourself up for not getting the extra 10%. We do this with others in catching them doing something wrong and forgetting to catch them doing something right.

All or nothing - When you see something as black or white no middle ground. Eg Similar to filtering, that mock test – you go as far as saying 'theres no point me even taking the test if I don't get 100%.' We also forget that the process has as much value as the result.

Blowing things out of proportion - When small problems become major disasters eg After answering a question wrong in class you may feel like you are a failure and no one will like you..

Labeling - Talking to yourself in a negative or critical way. Eg Miss a goal at a football match, and you call yourself an idiot or a loser

Fortune telling - You think you know what the future holds, and it's not good. This leads to feelings of hopelessness. Eg I'm never going to find the right girl, I'm too shy…

Facing negative thinking is really important. It's great to write them down but you don't have to do thought recording on paper, you can do it in the notes section of your phone, when you get really good at it, you can do it in your head.

Dentist scenario: *The Dentist says I need a filling….*

*What if the anaesthetic doesn't work and I feel it? What if I can't breathe, what if I swallow my tongue…. Thinking about these emotions I can label then **"scared emotions".***

***"100% fair and realistic thoughts are";** This dentist will do this procedure at least once a day, she's qualified, what about the thousands of people across the UK who are laying back with their mouths open just like me right now…*

*Breathe through my nose, calmly…**begin to calm my emotions.***

Anxiety is when we; worry excessively, experience panic attacks,

feel fearfully , lose sleep of experience insomnia.

With anxiety, we might experience;

- Racing heart

- Sweaty palms

- Shortness of breath

- Irritability

- Feeling like you are on the edge

Anxiety can also be experienced like a gremlin on your shoulder; like a bully making you fearful Taking control of the bully can help reduce the size of the gremlin.

Anxiety can also be experienced like a rainbow. Each colour is like a different anxiety eg panic, phobias, OCD, health anxieties.

Experts tell us R.E.D. can help anxiety:

<u>R</u>elaxation -including mindfulness in the moment, using breathing techniques eg Relax Plus app download for smart phones

<u>E</u>xercise – clears the mind and produces endorphins

<u>D</u>istraction – breaking cycle by being creative eg adult colouring, watching good films.

Lily Jo helps young people use the Worry Tree (next page) to think scenarios, like the ones below:

1: a loved one is diagnosed with a serious illness

2: You've ran up a massive phone bill that your parents don't yet know about

3: You've been getting close to your friend's girlfriend, you've started to have feelings for her…

THE WORRY TREE

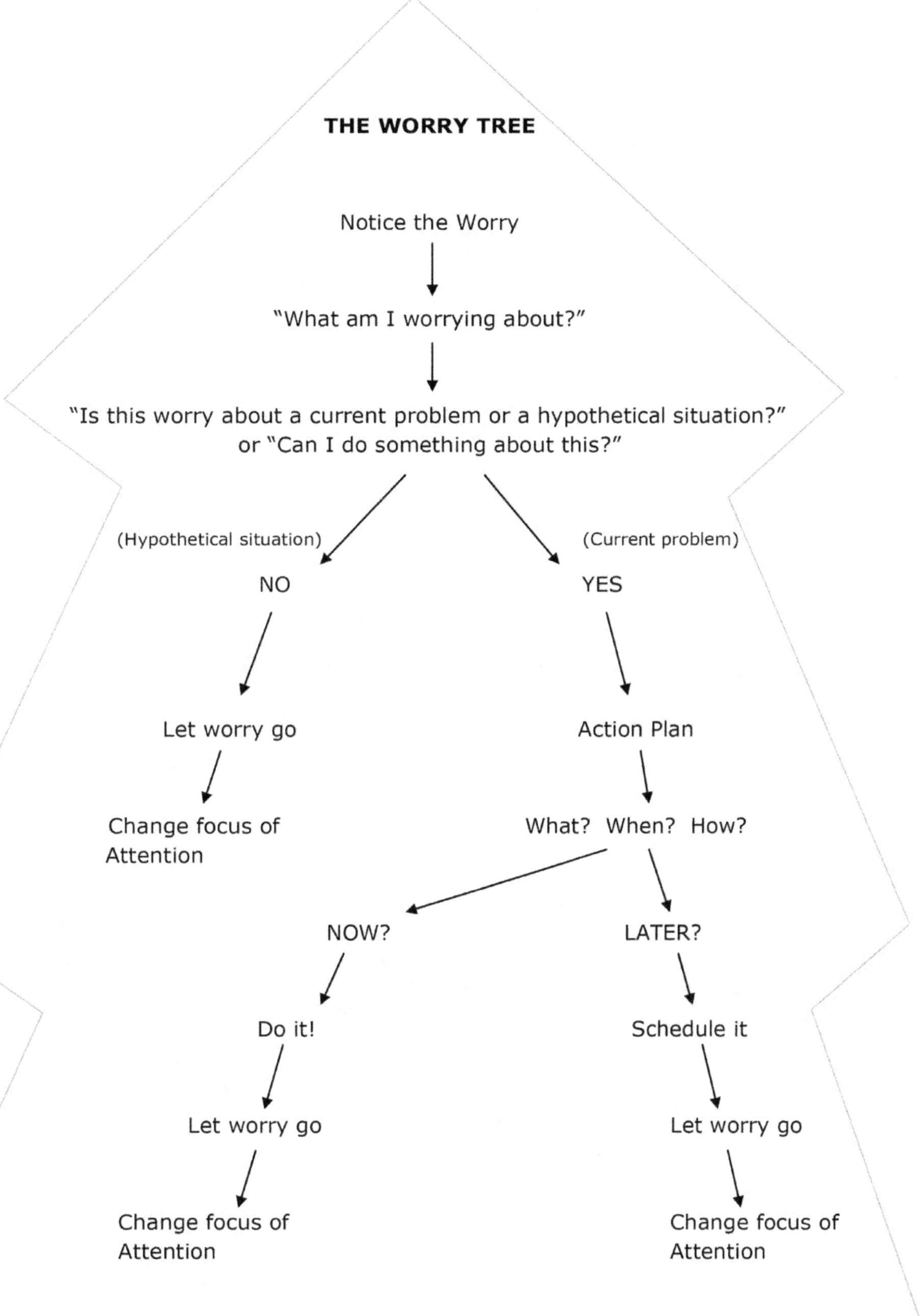

Life balance

Happiness = someone to love, a job to do and something to look forward to.

A definition of happiness can be helpful in providing some specific things to seek. We can begin to create a plan, put actions in to our diaries that move us forward on the journey.

Happiness = W L P G

Other experts have described happiness as a balance of **WLPG**: **W** is our work, **L** is living and is about how we feel about our life, **P** is playing and **G** is giving. The WLPG survey helps us see how we score ourselves in these areas and provides some opportunity to think about how to develop and improve these areas. We also believe it is beneficial to think about how you can grow these areas by getting them to overlap. Eg How can I bring more play and fun into my workplace.

Life balance can often feel like juggling balls or spinning plates or at best trying to balance the seesaw. But a more helpful image of life balance is cycling a bike. It not only involves balance, but it involves moving forward.

It requires concentration to get going and extra effort when we face steep hills. But it opens up a journey that can be transforming and create a legacy.

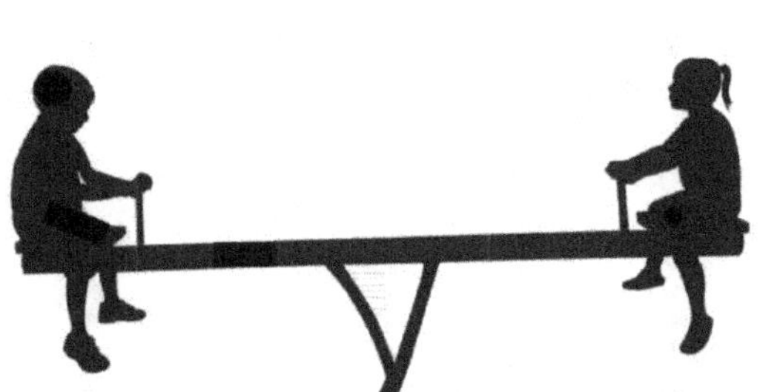
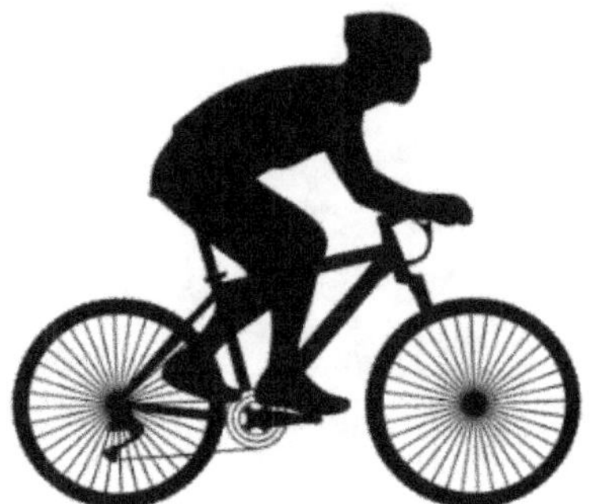

This image of a bicycle is more attractive to employers too, who pay staff to move things forward in an organisation. James Kerr in his book Legacy, describes the culture shift in the New Zealand All Blacks team that made them the best professional sports team in history. Legacy for them is not about personal glory but about "leaving the jersey in a better place". In other words, helping the team achieve now and after you've gone.

The All Blacks famously chant the Maori haka which reminds them of the sound of the *earthquake.* They acknowledge the challenge that faces them. They face a tumultuous event. They may die. But they also may come through it and live. Life is full of obstacles for all of us. But if we face them, with all our mind and all our heart, we can overcome them.

Life balance as WLPG

Life is made up of different dimensions: **Work; Living; Play; Giving**. Have a go at the WLPG questionnaire*, tick the boxes below and give yourself a score as to how you would rate each section of your life currently -5 is very high and 1 is very low.

W

REALISING POTENTIAL How well does your school work allow you to utilise your talents, gifts? How well does your school work enable you to live out your deepest values or your faith?

1 - 2 - 3 - 4 - 5

FULFILLING AND FUN Do you enjoy your school work and are you passionate about it?

1 - 2 - 3 - 4 - 5

RECOGNITION AND REWARD Do you feel you are well rewarded for your work? (extrinsically & intrinsically)

1 - 2 - 3 - 4 - 5

L

PERSONAL GROWTH How good do you feel about yourself, and your development as a person?

1 - 2 - 3 - 4 - 5

SENSE OF PURPOSE How well do your values and purpose in your life relate to the well-being of yourself and of others near and far?

1 - 2 - 3 - 4 - 5

EMPLOYABILITY Do you have the right mix of skills and experience to meet any future work/study challenge?

1 - 2 - 3 - 4 - 5

P

PERSONAL WELL-BEING Are you allowing yourself enough time to rest/relax? How much quality time and commitment are you giving to growing your well-being (and spiritual life).

1 - 2 - 3 - 4 - 5

INTERESTS Do you give enough time to hobbies, sports or leisure activities that are sources of pleasure?

1 - 2 - 3 - 4 - 5

SOCIAL LIFE Are you giving and receiving enough help, friendship, support, love and encouragement?

1 - 2 - 3 - 4 - 5

G

FRIENDS AND FAMILY Are you giving enough quality time, love, resources, help, friendship, support and encouragement to your close family and friends?

1 - 2 - 3 - 4 - 5

COMMUNITY AND ENVIRONMENT How much are you giving to improve your wider community? How much are you giving of your talents and skills for those less fortunate?

1 - 2 - 3 - 4 - 5

UNCONDITIONAL GENEROSITY How much do you give to people and projects at home and abroad, particularly where you expect no reward or return?

1 - 2 - 3 - 4 - 5

When completed, consider: Where do you score highly? Are there areas for development? What are the problems and barriers that need to be addressed? Do you see possible solutions and what are your intentions?

Further work: Consider whether there is any overlap of WLPG by drawing each as a circle that intersects with the other WLPG dimensions.

*acknowledgements to www.windmillsonline.co.uk

5 things

Moving forward and leaving a legacy involves learning some skills and building some confidence. Here are five things that experts agree are key to becoming more effective, whatever your age.

1. **Have a bigger yes!**

   Teenagers often struggle with FOMO (the fear of missing out), which causes them to thrill seek in ways that are destructive to wellbeing. The best way to delay gratification is to have a bigger yes. Thrill seeking is a natural desire of teenagers to reach out of their comfort zone, but there are healthy ways to do it. For example, rock climbing and overnight bivouacking or an organised trip to Africa that takes them out of their comfort zone

   Finding the "bigger yes" is best done by trying to take a birds eye view of your life; perspectives that enable you to look at your whole life span, rather than 3-5yrs goals, 1yr goals or current actions, projects and commitments which are lower level more detailed perspectives. Some personalities find it harder than others to see the big view. Getting alongside someone who is older and has lengthy experience in an area of interest is a really helpful way to get the birds eye view.

2. **Learn to say no.**

If we're going to achieve our bigger yes, then we need to learn to say no. It's important because we are bombarded by around 7,500 adverts per day all marketing to you trying to persuade you to say YES. Option paralysis is a real condition where we can't decide because we have so many choices. A study found that reducing the number of different jams on sale in a supermarket actually increased sales!   Delaying gratification is one of the developments of maturity, from child to adult. It involves learning to say "no, not now." Something else is at stake and is a higher priority to say yes to. Practical steps that can help include;

i) establish policies eg I'm in bed by 10pm

ii) delay giving an answer when invited to do something with others, giving yourself time to think carefully under less pressure, and communicate effectively your decision.

3. **Sweat the small stuff**

Whilst there is a self-help book out there called "Don't sweat the small stuff", experts say that sweating the right small stuff is important. It involves the practices of remembering names, key dates and getting back to people by phone or email.   It's this back end stuff that has power. Because its where integrity of character is seen and valued. It strengthens relationships by building trust and it translates into cash value in business.

4. **Stop trying to remember things**

Computers have two types of memory: A hard-drive for storing data and RAM drive for processing.   Your brain is much more like a RAM drive than a hard -drive. PCs crash when RAM is overloaded and so do people! To avoid a crash, learn to process incoming data. Capture it anyway you can. Top CEOs still use

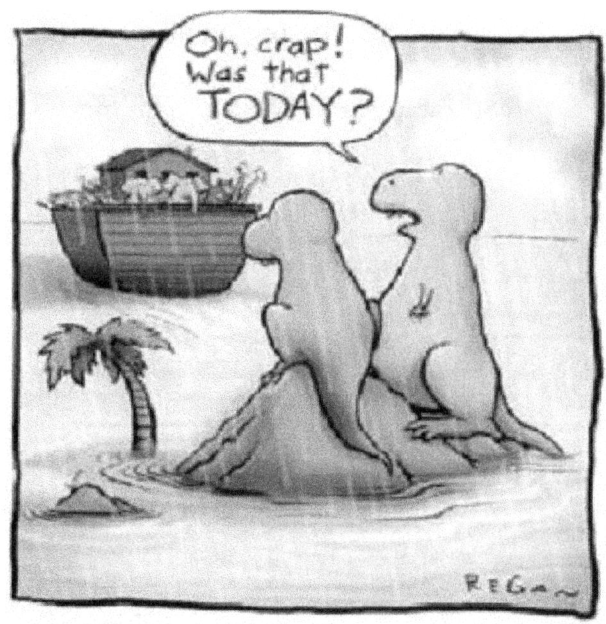

post-it notes, sticking them on to their "Today" folder as they walk from meeting to meeting. Then, when you have a moment, go through the captured items and process them by filing, deleting or actioning them now.

5. **Schedule everything**

Whether it's the rubbish bins to go out Wednesday night, a revision timetable, skyping a friend monthly to stay in touch. Get it in a diary or calendar format

6. **Develop routines**

Saying to yourself before you leave the house everyday "Keys, wallet, phone" is an excellent way to avoid being locked out or stuck later in the day. Making your sandwiches the night before saves money and helps make getting out on time in the morning.

Taking revision breaks really works to keep your mind fresh and productive. It's true that every hour of sleep before midnight is worth two after midnight. There are all sorts of routines that

you can create to help you be more effective.

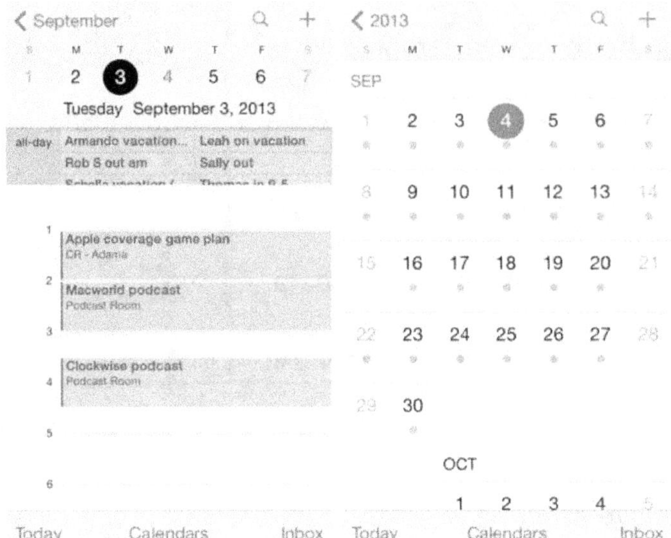

Schools: Spiritual wellbeing

Third Space Bolton believes all young people should have **an opportunity to choose a belief in God**. R.E lessons at school are a helpful introduction, but choosing a belief in God involves trying it out in the way that swimming involves getting into the water.

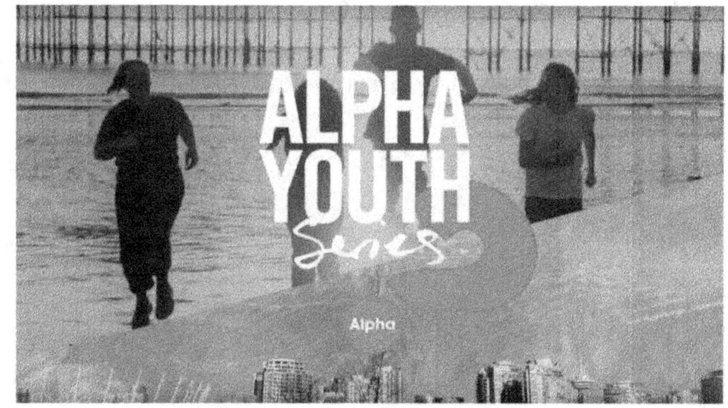

Third Space Bolton offers faith exploration for young people, often done during a lunch club.

Youth Alpha is an interactive series (13 episodes over 9 weeks) exploring the basics of the Christian faith. It can be previewed online at www.alpha.org/alpha-youth-series/

Big Bible Story is an interactive series produced by Third Space Bolton that explores the Bible, broken down into six sections: Creation, Fall, Israel, Jesus, Church, New Creation.

Fit4Life is an interactive series produced by Third Space Bolton which explores how we apply some the Bible's teaching on wellbeing into practice in our lives.

Unbelievable is an interactive series produced by Third Space Bolton that explores the debate about the compatibility of science and faith.

Faith based assemblies are offered which provide worship opportunities for young people.

Third Space Bolton partners with **Axia and Youth Unite,** two youth worship initiatives that draw young people from churches and high schools from across Farnworth and Bolton respectively.

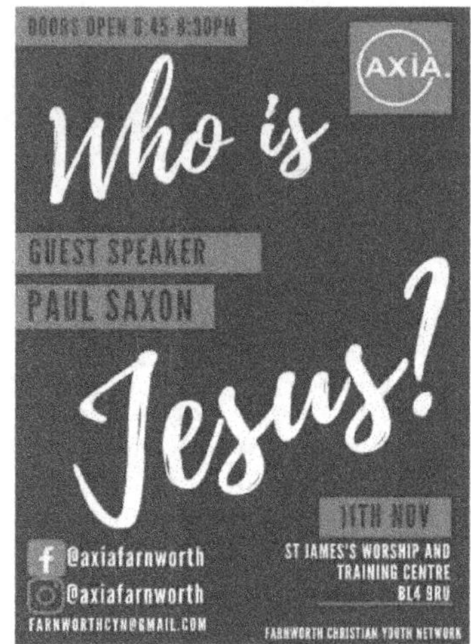

Cohesion is something that is worked for in Bolton. Third Space Bolton believes diversity is our strength and good relationships between ethnicities and religions is an important foundation for the wellbeing of a town. Third Space Bolton is committed to intentionally strengthening cohesion in Bolton. One of the ways we do this is by teaching peacemaking which unites us— a life skill for family life, school life and community life. This has been especially important after the Manchester Arena bombing. Approximately ten children from each high school across Greater Manchester were present at the Ariana Grande concert that night.

Student Linkup is a ministry provided by FusionMovement.org to help students connect to a church at university.

23% of students who go to church at home linkup with a church at university. This improves to over 90% where students participate in a Student Preparation Course before they go away.

Student Linkup Sessions: Bolton

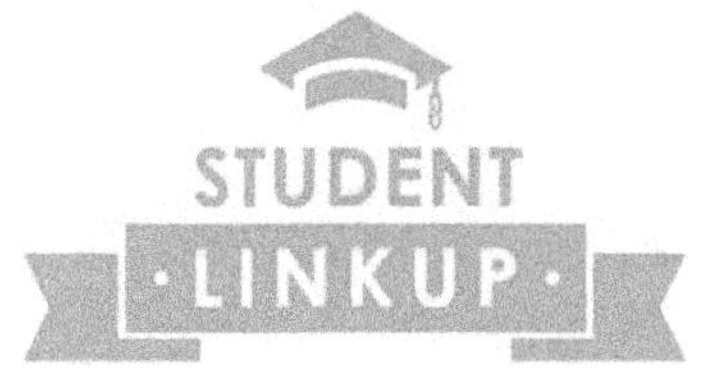

Off to University...

We want to help university students come to know Jesus and commit to being part of his family – the Church. If you are just starting university or already a student download the Student Linkup app to find the church for you.

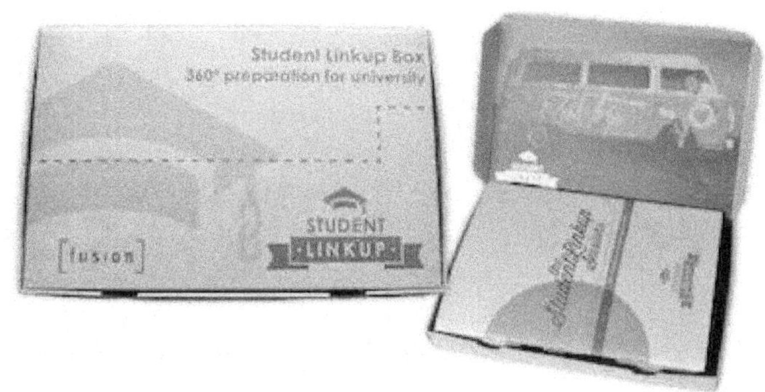

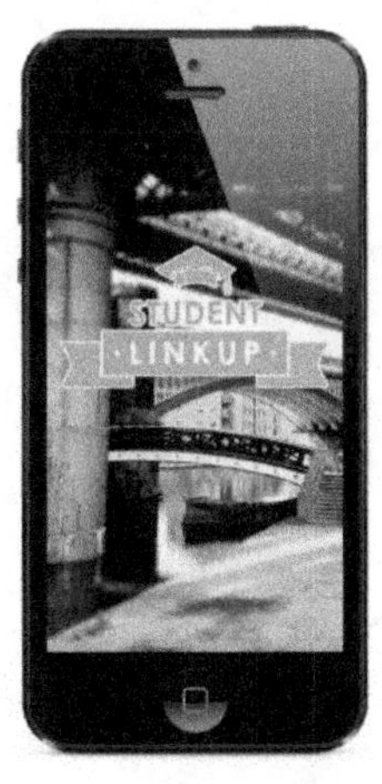

01. UNIVERSITY –THE START
    Combating anxieties and building confidence
02. UNIVERSITY –THE CULTURE
    Eyes wide open to student culture
03. UNIVERSITY –THE OPPORTUNITIES
    Choosing wisely
04. UNIVERSITY –THE LEGACY
    Three years and a whole life

Preparation

The Student Linkup Sessions are a 4 part student preparation course using the tool kit box (pictured above).   We'll also introduce you to the Student Linkup App which makes connecting with churches so much easier.

In Bolton, we'll be gathering together 6th formers who are planning to go to university or College.   We'll meet at Third Space Cafe over a luxury hot chocolate, discuss the sessions together and grill a university student to get an inside perspective.

4 Tuesday nights at 8pm in June.

Contact: office@thirdspacebolton.com
Third Space Cafe, 133 Deansgate, Bolton, BL1 1HA

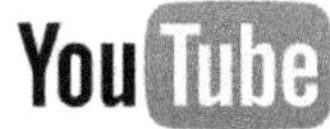
Student Linkup Sessions

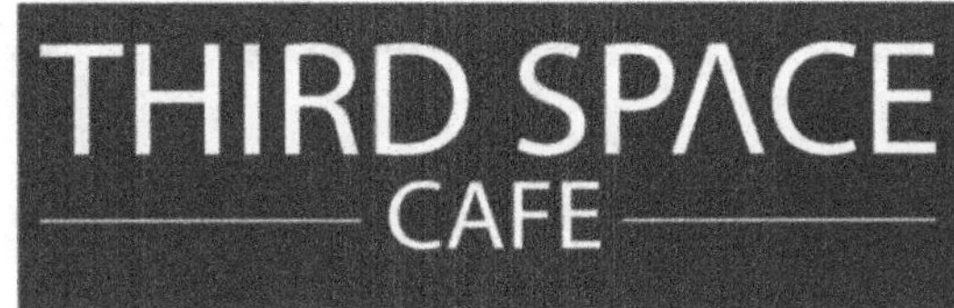

We're passionate about coffee…

…the aroma, the taste, it's cultural character and the conversation we enjoy with it.

At Third Space our pride and joy is our classic top quality steam espresso coffee machine built to the highest standards using the finest stainless steel, copper and brass. But add to that, the best tasting coffee from a fanatical coffee merchant with an ethical addiction, and we guarantee to serve you something special.

But there's more. Third space is a sociological term used to describe leisure time and at least one big coffee shop chain aims to be people's first choice for third space time. Third space is actually really important for people as it provides a time to rest and reflect on all of life, including your first space which is your family time and your second space, which is your work time. The Third Space Café aims to create space for customers and staff to learn and put into practice skills for wellbeing in the whole of their lives.

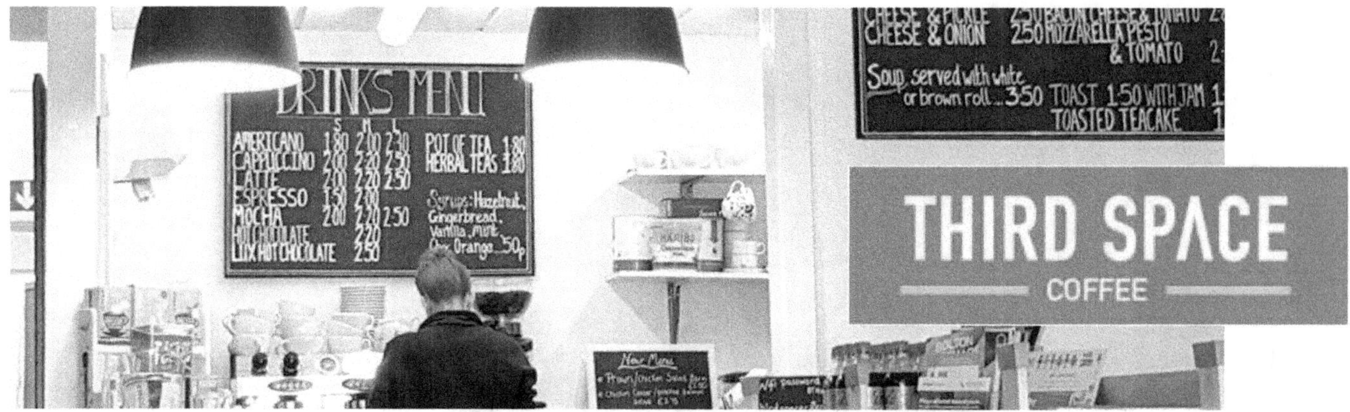

Education, Education, Education

"Leading employers prefer and value work experience over grades"

The Independent Newspaper

Work has the potential to enable us to flourish as human beings but it can also be a source of obstacles to our wellbeing. The Third Space Community Cafe provides tailored work experience placements where young people can be helped to develop skills, character and wellbeing through work experience.

Our specialised approach supports young people in overcoming common obstacles;

- **Emotional intelligence (EI) is understood to be a better predictor of success in job performance than IQ and there is a need to provide much more support and resources for this area of development and learning.**

  Adolescence is the third of six extraordinary human life stages and is the transition into adulthood. However, brain development in young people does not mature until the early twenties. The parts of the brain responsible for controlling impulses and planning ahead are along the last to develop. We know that EI is caught from role models more than it can be taught in the classroom. The café provides a great variety of social experiences with customers, staff and suppliers that help shape EI.

- **25% of young people suffer from emotional, behavioral and mental health problems that can be diagnosed.**

  Work experience placements at Third Space Community Cafe which offer coaching, education and a positive work environment are helping young people significantly improve their health and wellbeing.

Here's some of the testimonies from people connecting with the Third Space Café:

*"You not only inspire people to obtain personal achievements, you help them find work, ask pertinent questions, which I personally can also relate to which is why I so love to be on the sidelines of your meetings, **it reminds me of why I wanted to get better**. So carry on with your amazing support."*[1]

"I'm incredibly thankful to all at Third Space for their help and support for me. A year ago I was suffering from anxiety and depression finding it hard to leave the house and feeling very isolated. Today, I've discovered friends who have taught me

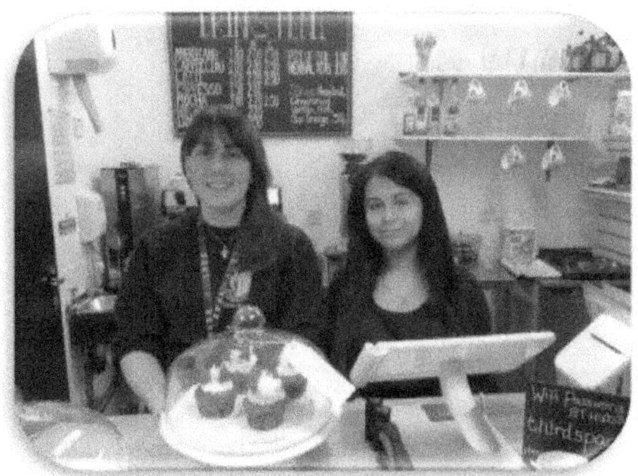

---

[1] Karen Ashton, customer of Third Space Cafe, commenting on Guy Hampson's leadership of the Fat2Fit project and the Fit4Life group, 2018.

*loads about myself and helped me improve my self confidence and life skills. **My life is truly different**.*"[2]

*"Third Space Cafe is **a very special place for me**. I would recommend it to anyone wanting to do work experience."*[3]

*"I became very low and had actually planned my suicide, thinking my wife and three girls would have a better life without me. But, on the day I planned to carry out my suicide, I was invited to volunteer at the Third Space Cafe project... **Third Space honestly saved my life**. It helped me return to a right mind and me and my family will forever be in debt to Third Space."*[4]

"The Third Space Community Café have provided excellent work placement opportunities for learners with varying support needs. They provide a supportive learning environment to develop valuable practical and personal skills. Their person centred approach has been very successful in enabling our learners to equip themselves to progress their lives."[5]

---

[2] Ash Crook, age 29, volunteer at Third Space Cafe
[3] Reece, Autism special needs, age 21.
[4] Yomi Aminu, age 35, Nigerian asylum seeker living in Britain.
[5] Gary Mangan, Employment Placement Officer, Bolton College

Work Experience at Third Space Cafe

- **Come and check us out at Third Space Coffee.** We are at 133 Deansgate , Bolton, BL1 1HA. Come and visit to see where we are and perhaps try our coffee or our delicious milkshakes.

- **Contact Julie Regan our Cafe Manager** on 01204 384 233 or by email- office@thirdspacebolton.com. She can tell you more and answer any questions you may have.

- **Complete a Third Space Work Experience Registration Form** This helps us to discuss a work experience placement with you. We will explain and give you a sheet that tells you what you can expect from us, for example, how we will support your development and how often you will meet for reviews of your placement.

- **Get fantastic experience.** Learn about catering in the food and drink industry and equip yourself for paid jobs.

  - **Barista Training.** "Coffee is becoming like wine –people want to learn how to taste it, where it's from, how it's made".

  - **Food and Hygiene.** Learn about what's required to open your doors for business and achieve the Level 1 Food Hygiene qualification.

  - **Learn skills to help you run a business.** Get valuable teamwork experience and learn about interviews, managing people, money, stock, regulations, marketing and social media with input from local experts which will help equip you for success.

- **There's more to you!** One of the reasons "leading employers prefer and value work experience over grades" is that the workplace really develops your work and life skills. Work experience can give you a reference that shows how you get on with your boss, your team and your customers. We will give you opportunities to learn work skills and accelerate the growth of your character. Young people love our Fit4Life discussions which develop the work and life skills of self-awareness, a valuable foundation in building character and understanding yourself and others.

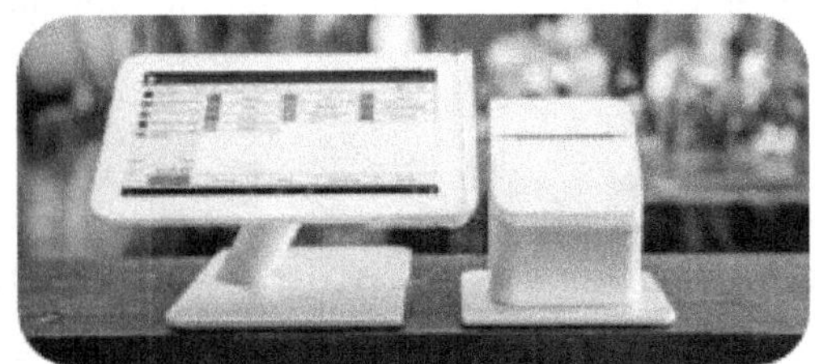

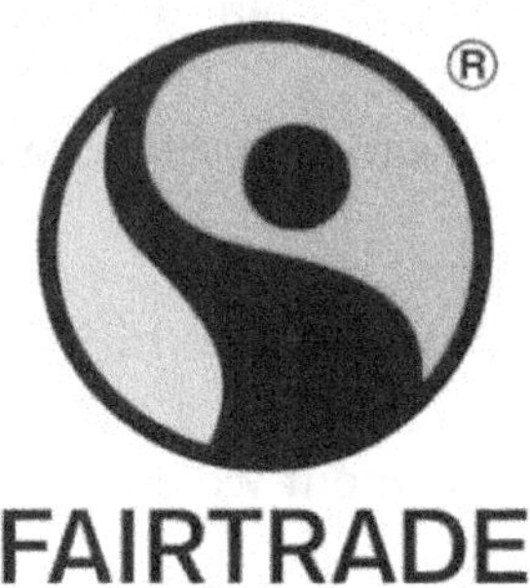

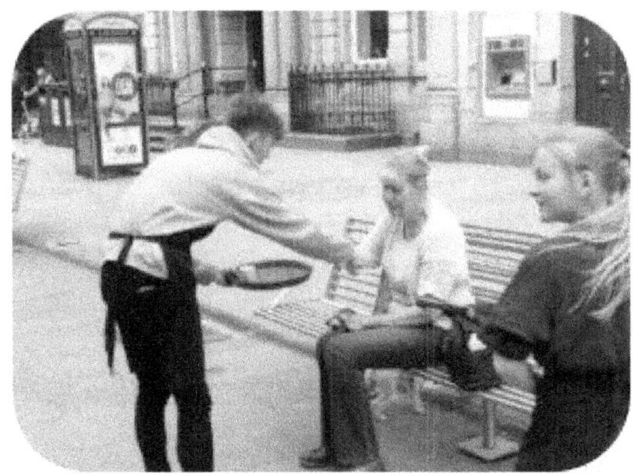

Measurement:

"Give me a stock clerk with a goal and I'll give you a man who will make history. Give me a man with no goals and I'll give you a stock clerk."

JC Penny (Founder of Penny Stores USA)

"By looking at your diary this week it is possible to predict where you will be in 3-5 years' time -the idea that our big goals are made up of lots of small goals that we have to be committed to."

Setting goals and reviewing them is crucial to progress. Third Space Café aims to do this not only for job performance but for wellbeing as well. Our client reporting pack includes;

1.) Client registration form

2.) Client review form -including signposting

3.) Work experience record recording completed work tasks

4.) Five Ways to Wellbeing (over the page)- an evidence-based public mental health survey, which aims to improve mental health and wellbeing. Working alongside someone gives our coaches a great opportunity to see the whole person; skills, confidences, character and wellbeing.

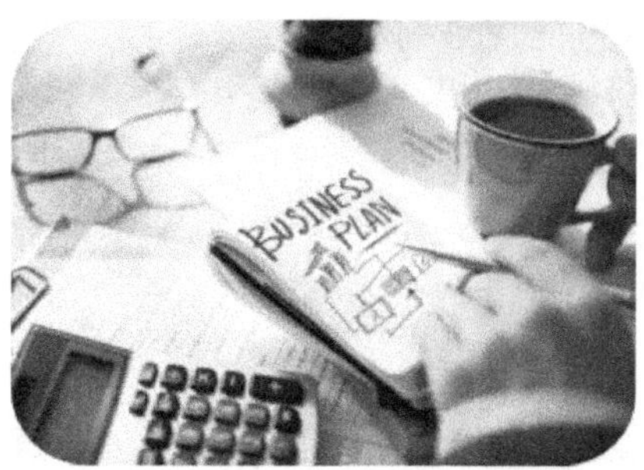

Name:_________________________   Age:_________

Date:_________________________   Gender:_________

0 1 2 3 4 5 6 7 8 9 10

1. Would you like to learn new skills?

0 1 2 3 4 5 6 7 8 9 10

2. Have you volunteered before?

0 1 2 3 4 5 6 7 8 9 10

3. How easy do you find it is getting to know and talking to people?

0 1 2 3 4 5 6 7 8 9 10

4. How aware are you of other people's feelings?

0 1 2 3 4 5 6 7 8 9 10

5. Do you exercise?

0 1 2 3 4 5 6 7 8 9 10

6. How well do you sleep?

7. Have you got family and friends that can support you? 0 1 2 3 4 5 6 7 8 9 10

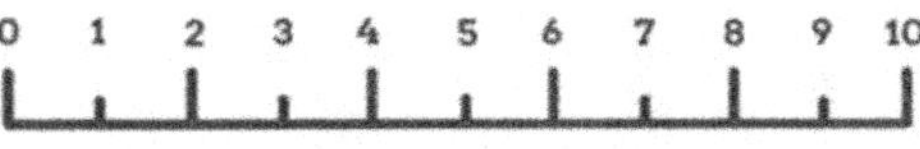

8. Do you have any money worries?

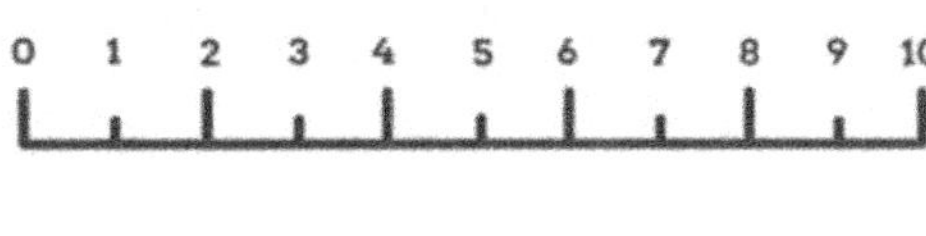

0 1 2 3 4 5 6 7 8 9 10

9. Do you feel anxious some times?

0 1 2 3 4 5 6 7 8 9 10

10. Do you find managing your symptoms and medication ok?

0 1 2 3 4 5 6 7 8 9 10

11. Have you any medical issues?

12. Are there any triggers you want to tell us?

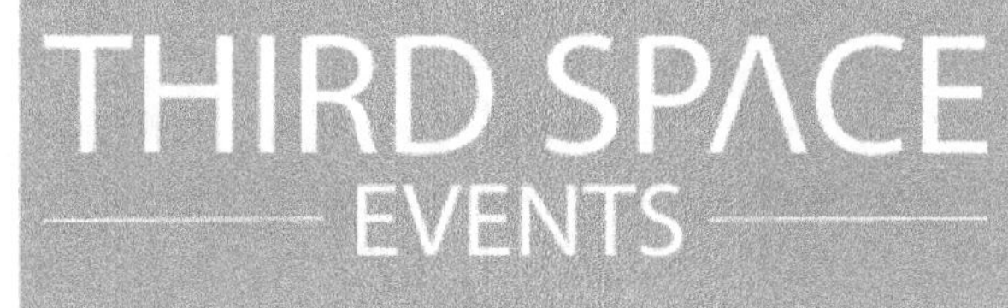

Gather, Grow, Give

The Christian tradition has, over the centuries, found a pattern of community that offers moral purpose, is fulfilling and delivers a legacy. That pattern involves "gathering, growing and giving" and it's the structure behind Third Space Events.

Gathering: People need social events that bring them together with others and enable stronger relationships. The leader of these events is hugely important, acting as the social architect of the gathering.

Third Space Events have collaborated with Bolton Wanderer's Community Trust in recent years to run an event called Family Faith Football at the Bolton Wanderer's stadium, four or five times a season. Third Space Events help plan and lead the FFF event, manage the finances and invite Third Space clients to attend (often subsidising their tickets). These pre-match all age events use a football theme to explore wellbeing, using football pundits, a football focus and interactive activities in one of the best hospitality suites at the club.

Third Space Events experiences a demand from the community eg to host the Bolton Miscarriage Group, at the Café every month, to support mothers who have are dealing with the loss of not been able to carry a child to full term.

Many ad hoc events are run throughout the year, including Caring for Ex-offenders seasonal meals, Open Mic nights, Silent Discos, Bolton Church Leaders meetings and many others.

Growing: Integral to wellbeing is the feeling that we are growing and Third Space Events is proud to work with people with different needs.

Fat2Fit is a complex needs men's group that meets weekly and helps men to lose weight by a combination of exercise and better eating. It is a strongly relational group and additional pastoral care is offered as it's required during the week.

The Bolton Discipleship Year has been run for the last five years, training over fifty Christian young adults in theology, ministry and leadership one day a week whilst they are on one year training placements in local churches or charities. Many of the graduates of this programme have stayed in Bolton and serve their communities as inspiring young leaders.

In January 2019, Third Space Bolton launched the Fit4Life at Work Course in partnership with the Town Centre Chaplain. This is a six to ten week course that enables workers in the town centre to come the Third Space Café for lunch and be involved in a discussion group about developing wellbeing in the workplace.

Giving: Every summer we run and invite clients and friends to run the Manchester 10K with us to raise money for good causes. In 2016 Bolton Wanderer's Community Trust joined in with us to create an entry of nearly one hundred runners from our community. We have also worked with schools to get them to run the 10K or Juniors run.

On Monday's we advertise the Café as a Dementia Friendly venue, offering specialist support for sufferers and carers, enabling a normalised experience for those who might otherwise be put off from going out. This inter-generational contact is a positive experience at Third Space Café and as it develops we will add specific activities, partnering with other Dementia Friendly organisations such as the Octagon Theatre and Precious Memories.

Churches across Bolton are aware that students going away to university for the first time often find it hard to connect with a new church. Third Space Events works with local churches to host the Student Link Up Course at the Café. This course increases the chances of students linking up with churches that can support them in a new town from 30% to over 90%.

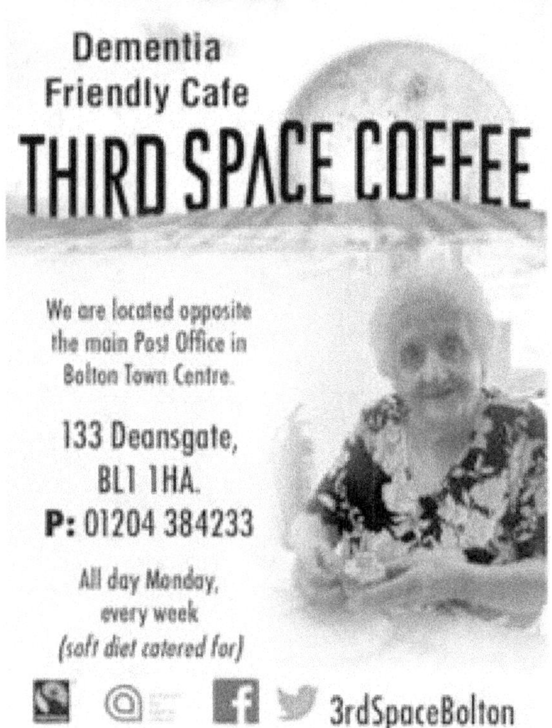

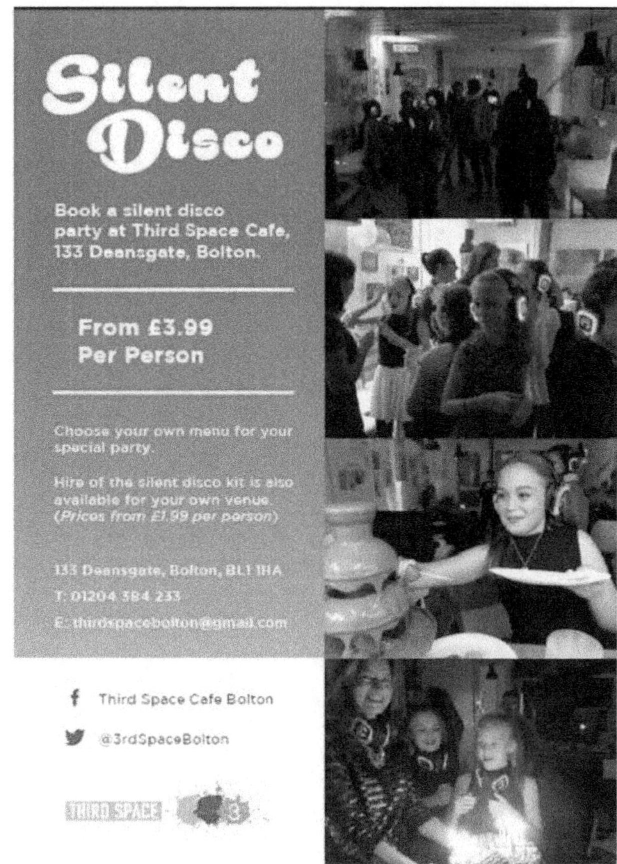

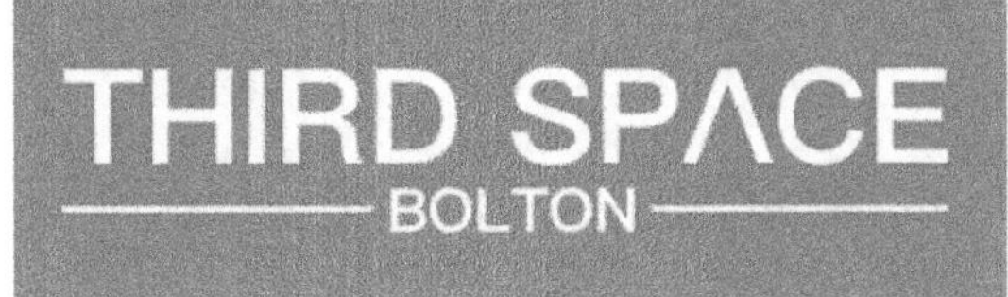

Sustainability

Third Space Bolton was founded in September 2015, when the Bishop of Bolton opened the café and launched the schools and events team. We were visited by the Mayor of Bolton who commended our work and we now have some of the biggest Bolton brands as clients.

Bolton Council Community and Voluntary Sector have encouraged Third Space since we started at the time of writing are now supported for two years by their Health and Wellbeing funding.

Bolton School Boys and Girls division, an outstanding independent school, is our biggest school client. Heather Tunstall (Head of 6th Form) says;

"We are happy working with Third Space as part of our 6th form enrichment programme. Their

flexible approach allows us to work together to design sessions that suit our needs and their speakers are engaging and professional in their approach."

Bolton Wanderer's Community Trust fund a weekly young adult men's group hosted in the café and run by our events team, delivering life coaching. Stephen Thomas (Bolton Wanderer's Community Trust) says;

"We're delighted with the service that Third Space provides.

The numbers of young adults attending the café speaks for itself.

For many of them, this is their most important time of the week."

Bolton College have sent a number of their students for work experience. Gary Mangan (Employment Placement Officer, Bolton College) says;

"The Third Space Community Café have provided excellent work placement opportunities for learners with varying support needs. They provide a supportive learning environment to develop valuable practical and personal skills. Their person-centred approach has been very successful in enabling our learners to equip themselves to progress their lives."

Bolton young people are at the centre of all our work and are invited and consulted to lead and guide our work.

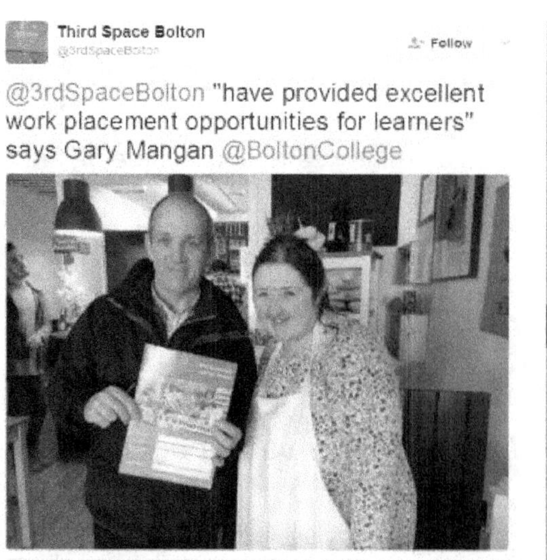

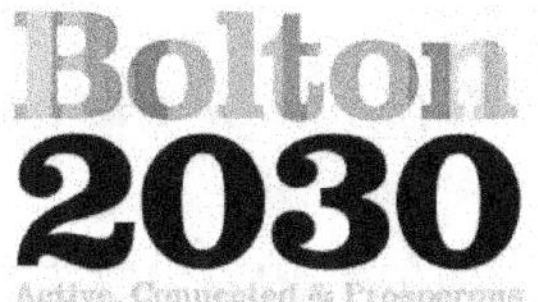

Partnership

Third Space Bolton is a partner of Bolton 2030

Bolton 2030 is a Vision Partnership connecting the Public, Private and Third Sector together in a strategic partnership to make Bolton a better place to start well, live well and age well.

- More than 1 million people fall into destitution in the UK. People who lack heating, food or are homeless and feel without hope.

- 25% people suffer from serious mental health problems

- Bolton is a city of sanctuary, receiving thousands of people seeking asylum and British citizenship

Church leaders in Bolton agreed that whilst churches do laudable work, they could be more strategic in joining up to have a greater impact on the big picture of the borough. Since 2016, church leaders from across the town have met regularly to pray and plan the church's response to Bolton 2030 called Passion Bolton 2030. This has resulted in four conferences to-date, each gathering around one hundred Christian leaders from across the town to connect and engage in a more joined up vision for Bolton.

We are not unique in Bolton. A city gospel movement is developing globally that seeks to be;

"unified by the gospel and vision to reach the city, growing the church faster than the population, in order to influence the city and bring social, cultural and spiritual transformation."

In Bolton, like many other places, we are engaged in a long-term conversation about the future of our town and the role the church has to play in God's transformation.

We want to see a borough-wide vision for the town (15 year monitorable vision)

-socially -debt, homelessness, isolation, aspiration, health, education, cohesion

-culturally -attitudes, morale, creativity

-spiritually -church planting, discipleship, leadership development

There must be:

-a unity across God's church in Bolton. Across traditions, BME, urban and suburban, key sphere leaders, the young, gender, class, church members and Christians organisations

-a partnership between private and public and third sectors

-a releasing of our people, validating their work, empowering, networking in key spheres

-prayer that sees outcomes of the body of Christ more unified, members of churches working together, the town improving culturally, socially, spiritually and the church growing and flourishing.

"The future will not be a new big tower of power. Our hope in the future is the hope into well-trodden paths from house to house. That is the image that holds a lot of promise for our future." Raimundo Panikkar

Finances

Third Space Bolton is a Charitable Incorporated Organisation 1163739 listed on the Charity Commission website.

We are grateful for a number of kick-start grants and giving that enabled us to set up, notably from the Andrew Christian Trust, the Lottery Awards for All and some generous individuals.

Our financial model has aimed to find funding for our work through four strands:

1.) Café trading with over the counter sales, rental bookings (39%)

2.) Trading with schools (3%)

3.) Grants from Trust Funds and from local health and social care awards (44%)

4.) Donations from individuals, businesses and churches (14%)

Our average annual expenditure has been £59,245. For every pound in cash spent, volunteers have given time in-kind worth approximately 55 pence.

In 2018, we invested £3K in a professional fundraising activity using Chell Fundraising which returned over £50,000 over two years. The Trustees take the view that we will continue to do this going forward to build sustainability.

We were also grateful for advice, training and support from Bolton Council Community and Voluntary Sector (CVS) which helped us sharpen our own applications for grant funding by articulating the need Third Space Bolton meets when filtered through the grant criteria – summarised by the following "Three Steps diagram worked example.

A small but key investment in our website (www.thirdspacebolton.com) using the easy to use Word Press system improved our communications with the public and our stakeholders. We also benefitted from the coaching offered by the Christian organisation: www.the-message-works.org.uk

Step 1 - Define the Problem

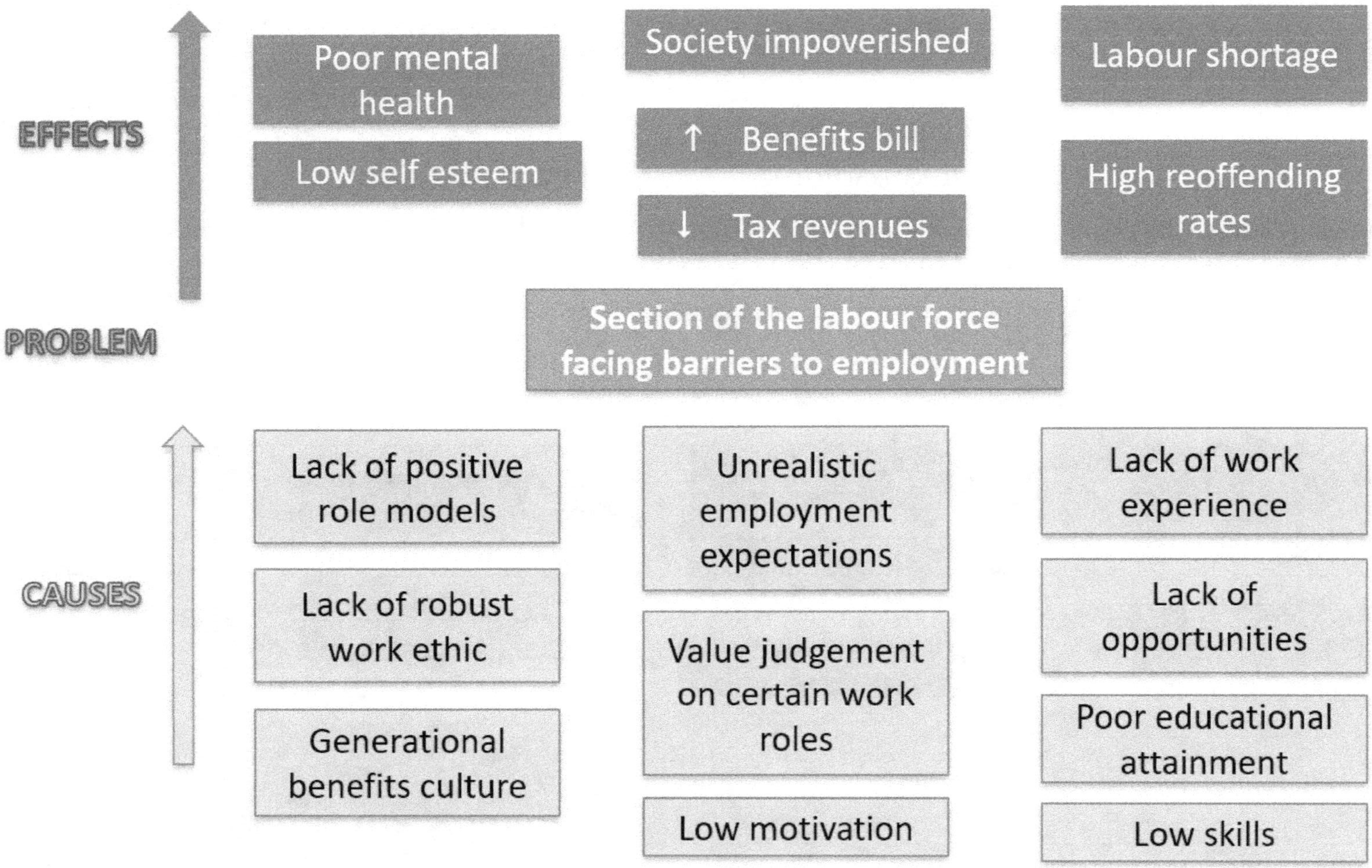

Step 2 - Define the Solution

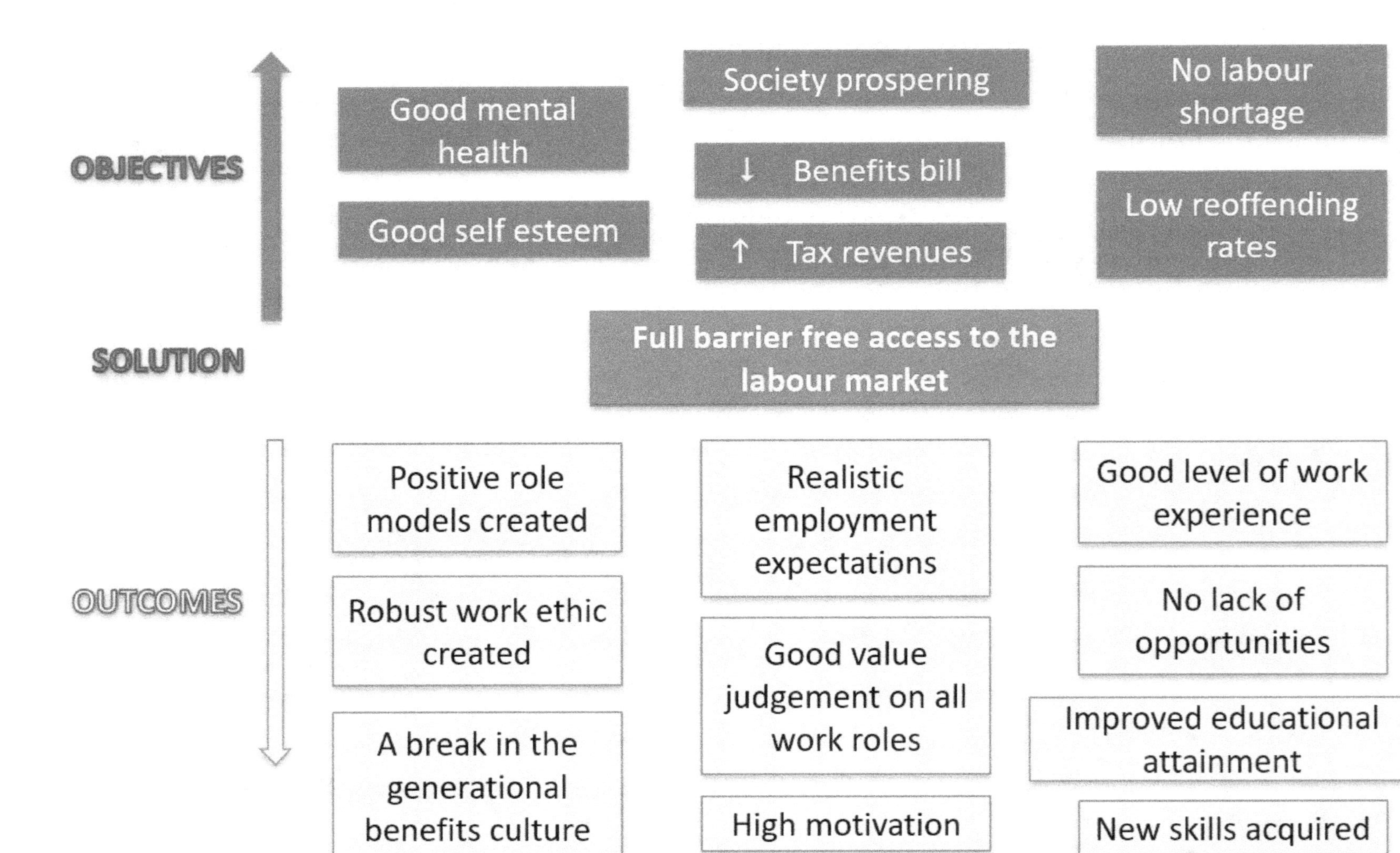

Step 3 - Define the Relationship

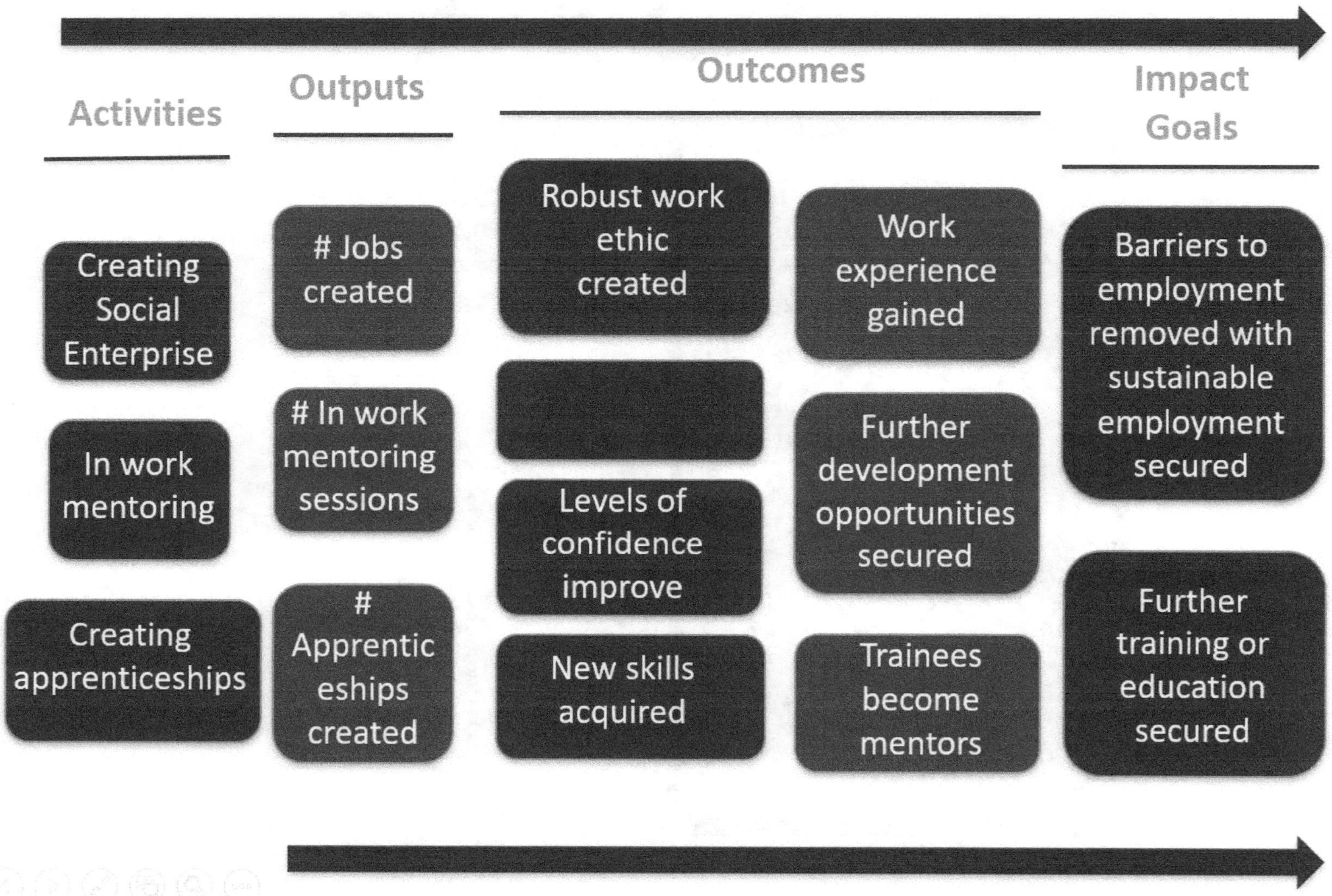

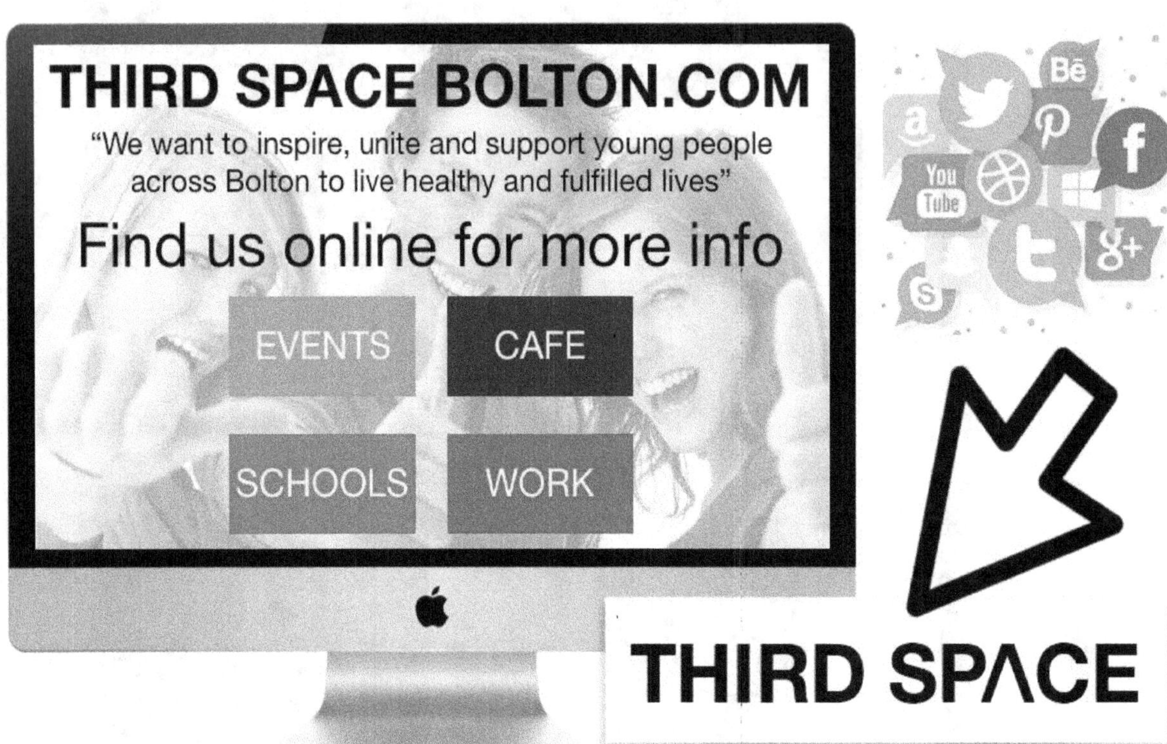

"**Health** is a state of complete physical, mental and social **well-being** and not merely the absence of disease or infirmity."
- World Health Organisation.

Let's carry on the conversation…
office@thirdspacebolton.com
07701089420

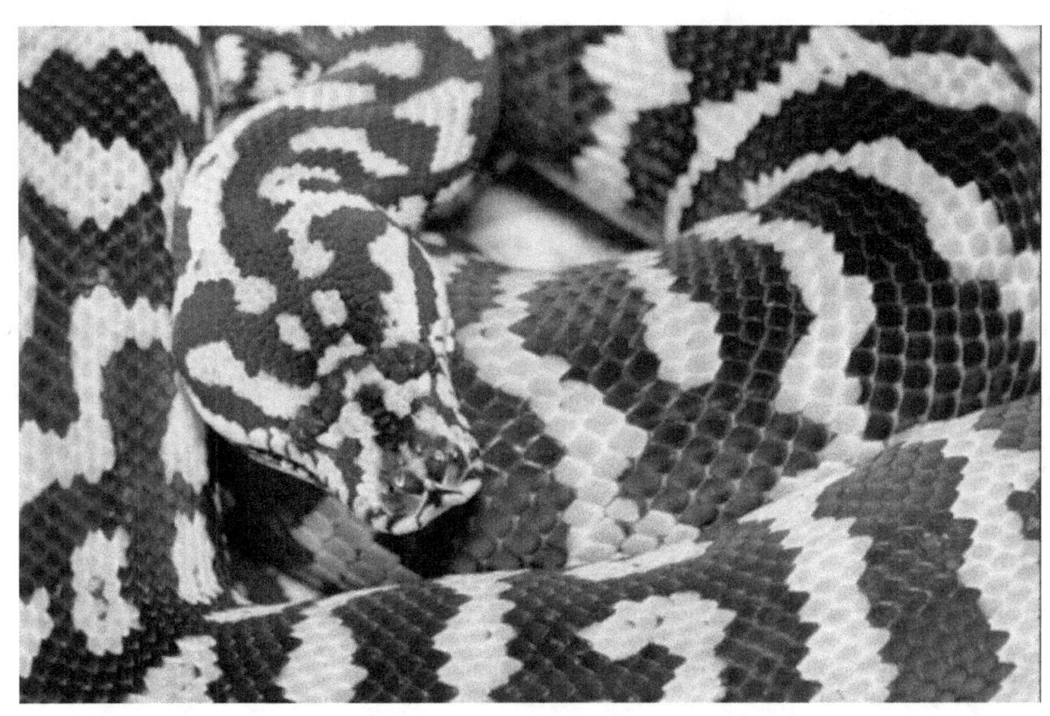

ABOUT THE AUTHOR

Mark Cowling is a Church of England minister working in Greater Manchester and is founder of Third Space Bolton, a charity supporting the wellbeing of young people. Other publications available on Amazon include Fit 4 Life Volumes 1, 2 and 3.

All profits from the sales of this book will be given to the work of reaching out to young people in Christian ministry.